Be Iconic:

Healthy and Sexy at Any Age

How to Be "Nose to Toes" Fabulous for the Rest

of Your Life

Eudene Harry, MD, author of *Anxiety 101*

ISBN: 1719378649
ISBN 13: 978-1719378642

Table of Contents

Chapter 1:

Defining Sexy

I was once afraid of people saying, "Who does she think she is?"

Now, I have the courage to stand up and say, "This is who I am."

—Oprah Winfrey (*What I Know for Sure*)

Sexiness is acceptance of the fact that you are perfectly flawed.

Today, we find too many reasons to diminish ourselves, to not shine, and to not be the healthiest, happiest version of ourselves. We let others determine our worth and how we feel about ourselves. We then act according to their idea of us and not who we truly are. These others can be voices that you have carried from your childhood telling you that you are not enough—not thin enough, smart enough, and so on—or they may be voices or circumstances today, constantly pointing out areas that they feel are lacking. So you withdraw, bury your music, hide your light, and give away your power. You forfeit your right to be your best self, and it shows up in the extra weight you carry, the sleepless nights, the chronic illness, and your lack of joy and health. I wrote this book because I want to give you the power to take your life back and say, "I am more than you can ever imagine because what you call flaws are well-placed facets that when polished, will blind you with their brilliance. I am **#PerfectlyFlawed**."

When most of us think of being healthy and sexy, we may envision Kate Upton posing for the cover of *Sports Illustrated,* or Beyoncé gracing the cover of numerous magazines, or any one of the Victoria's Secret models during their sassy runway walk, or David Beckham on his latest "Sexiest Man Alive" *People* magazine photoshoot. We may then find ourselves comparing and negating everything we are or hope to be. I challenge you to stop, step back, and ask yourself this question: What, exactly, do I find appealing about these women and men?

At first, we may be tempted to immediately point out their physical attributes and features, but I ask you to take another, closer look. Let's look past the flat abs, the oiled muscles, and the windblown hair. What is it that you find mesmerizing? Are you drawn in by the confidence the Victoria's Secret models portray with the strut in their step? Does the glow in Beyoncé's skin that says, "I am happy, healthy, and active" create a twinge of longing for that sense of vibrancy you once had? Do you recognize that light that shines through her eyes and that smile that says, "I am happy with who I am and where I am?" Does that slight defiance in the tilt of her chin that says, "What you may think of me does not diminish me in any way," make you want to take a page from her book? I want you to consider that these may be the attributes you yearn to recognize in yourself. After all, I am sure you can think of individuals in your world with flat, defined, sculpted abdominal musculature and windblown hair who are not necessarily healthy, sexy, or happy.

So how then do I define *healthy* and *sexy*? Let's start with defining *health*. According to the World Health Organization's definition, *health* is "not only the absence of infirmity and disease but the presence of a state of physical, mental, and social well-being." In medicine and life today, we are very focused on the absence of infirmity and disease. When you go for your annual wellness checkup, you are screened for diseases like diabetes, hypertension, and, depending on age, cancers—all very appropriate but certainly not all-inclusive. Even if you were given a mini mental health evaluation or screening using the Patient Health Questionnaire (sample found at the end of the chapter), the goal is to identify depression, another illness. Again, this is appropriate. A wellness visit is not designed to identify health by looking for the presence of physical, mental, and social well-being; it is designed to identify the absence of disease and infirmity. This statement is in no way meant to disparage the system but rather to identify its limitations. Once you acknowledge the limitations, you are empowered to look elsewhere for solutions because now you realize that health is also the presence of physical, mental, and emotional well-being.

You can ask yourself, "Am I healthy? Physically, am I eating nutrient-dense foods? Am I paying attention to the amount of activity that my body requires to keep it a well-oiled machine? Am I surrounded by people and circumstances that help me grow and are supportive? Am I able to take life's stressors in stride? Are my thoughts fertilizers that nourish me as I grow into the person I want to be, or are they more like toxic sludge that I bathe in every day?"

Now that we have a better understanding of *healthy*, how do we define *sexy*? I have created an acronym that summarizes what *sexy* is to me:

- *S* for *self-confident*

- *E* for *energized*

- *X* for *x-ing negative self-talk*

- *Y* for *yourself, unapologetically*

When all of these components come together, the outcome is a self-confident, energetic person who is unapologetically present in each moment of his or her life—and that is sexy.

Merriam-Webster's Dictionary defines *sexy* as "generally attractive and interesting." I love the word *interesting*. Notice that the definition does not say a pretty face, symmetrical features, big eyes, or long legs but, rather, "interesting." I would go out on a limb and say that part of the reason many of us feel that we have lost our shine is that slowly, over the years, for whatever reason, we begin to lose interest not only in things and people around us but also—and more importantly—in ourselves. When was the last time you truly thought of yourself as "generally attractive, appealing, and interesting?" Accepting and relaxing into who you are allows you to refocus all the energy you spend suppressing your voice and being self-critical into excavating all the parts of you that truly make you shine. Imagine moving from an environment that constantly berates you for not being the perfect rendition of someone else to a supportive environment that recognizes and accepts the uniqueness that is you. That is the power of self-acceptance. You will walk a little taller, laugh a little louder, and exude the confidence that comes with being at ease in your own skin. Confidence, in my opinion, has always been an essential ingredient in the recipe for "sexy."

So, as you can see, "healthy" and "sexy" are inextricably intertwined, with each one highlighting the strength and the beauty of the other.

I hope this book takes you on a journey to discover—or, rather, to remember—how to illuminate your external beauty with the flattering light of self-acceptance, enhance it with the soft glow of health and well-being and accentuate it with the confidence of knowing how to bring out the best in you. When you put all of these together, who can resist the appealing flame that is you?

How Health and Sexiness Became My Business!

At this point, you might be thinking that I couldn't possibly understand the challenges you face on a daily basis. Let me assure you that the twenty-five years I have practiced medicine and my board certification in emergency medicine and integrative holistic medicine in no way exempts me from the challenges that life continues to present. I would like to think that on some level, I am you. In life, I assume many roles. I am a mother of two, wife, physician, employee, employer, business owner, entrepreneur, family therapist, peacekeeper in the home, cook, butler, and maid, to name a few. I am also a person concerned about my health and well-being, my stress levels, my children, my marriage, my business, the future of medicine, and the future of our country and the world. I am a person challenged every day with finding time, energy, and knowledge to do and be what I need to do and be that day.

I am a woman in my fifties who lives in the same society as you do—a society that sends us messages daily that getting older means you are no longer vibrant, attractive, or interesting. So, oftentimes, we find ourselves expending a large amount of energy on recreating the "us" that existed years ago. The issue is, we cannot duplicate the exact conditions of years past, nor should we want to do so. If we do so, then we are denying who we are now and missing the opportunity to celebrate and maximize the "us" of today. Saying no to who you are on a daily basis causes your light to begin to dim and your presence to diminish, so much so that you become a shadow of what you were meant to be. Society can then say, "See, who you are is not attractive, appealing, or interesting." But, in reality, you have not shown them who you are now.

I would like to challenge you to live every day embracing and nourishing the uniqueness that is you. In this vast world, there might be people who look like you or have traits that remind others of you, but there is always only just one you. We are always in search of something unique to show that we are special, when the truth is, we are already in possession of the most unique treasure we can ever hope to find—ourselves. Hopefully, the information in this book will help you use the past to propel you to develop your own unique plan to create the healthiest, sexiest you in the now.

Where Did My "Sexy" Go?

Odds are, your "sexy," or the things that make you uniquely you, did not completely disappear. Battered and worn, they may be seeking shelter underneath the surface, hiding from the daily influx of self-criticism that seems to seep through to the very essence of who you are, slowly stealing away confidence, joy, and even health. The true you is most likely waiting and searching for the smallest opportunity, the slightest hint of encouragement, or the tiniest glimpse of acceptance to start the process of shedding that veil of uncertainty, that cloak of doubt that has kept you from living the life you were meant to live.

So, picking up a book called *Healthy and Sexy at Any Age* might be the first clue that something is amiss. Perhaps you are beginning to realize that you may have made an unconscious decision some time ago that you are no longer entitled to feel vibrant or to live your life out loud. You may have unconsciously incorporated some arbitrary rule that society perpetuates, stating that if you are a certain age or weight or some other random marker, you should slink away into the shadows to make room for others. The truth is, your being less has never made anyone more; it has only made you less.

Of course, there could be many other reasons to feel that you have lost your sex appeal. I have listed a few reasons below:

- Health conditions
- Having/raising children
- Getting older, with all of its many physical and emotional changes
- Work/professional life
- Voices that you have carried with you all your life telling you that you are not enough
- Voices around you now working to convince you that you are lacking

- That small voice in your head that has become the champion for those people and situations that have sought, over the years, to belittle and erode your belief in yourself
- The general overwhelming "wear and tear" and stress of daily living

If we're not careful, our sense of self and sexiness can slowly slip away until, one day, we look in the mirror and simply do not recognize the person staring back at us. I ask you to keep in mind that the feelings of desirability and vitality you seek are not limited to youth and, in fact, can actually be enhanced by the experience of living. After all, Halle Berry, Jane Fonda, and my own mother are living examples that sexiness and vibrancy do not have an age or an expiration date.

That's why it's so critical to identify the qualities that define sexiness for you and to recognize and acknowledge these traits in yourself. Your "sexy" didn't disappear, but maybe your confidence did.

Healthy and Sexy at Any Age will help guide you from sexy hair and nose to healthy fingers and delectable toes, from luscious lips to sexy hips, and everything in between! It will also help you discover why a sharp, agile mind and a strong, healthy heart are just as important to getting your "sexy" back as hormonal balancing and stress management. So, follow me on this libido-liberating journey to unleashing the full power and potential that is you.

How Do I Know If I'm Sexy?

Before we move on to the brain where, believe it or not, all sexy starts, I want to bring a little perspective to the "Am I or am I not sexy?" conversation. So let's play a game.

You Might Be Sexy If...

- **You're confident:** One thing all of the sexy people I'm writing about have in common is, confidence, and confidence is always sexy.

- **You're enthusiastic:** When you are enthusiastic about life, it means you're eager, hungry, and ready to learn more, to enjoy more, and to participate more—and what can be sexier than that! Remember, sexiness is interesting.

- **You're mature:** George Clooney, Helen Mirren, and Sophia Loren are all over fifty and all exude an immense amount of sex appeal. We have to remember that wherever we are, at whatever stage of life we are, we cannot rewind the clock. Trying to do so means we are focusing on something in the past, perhaps to the detriment of the now. Why direct energy to a past that cannot be recaptured or changed when we can take that same energy and harness it to unleash the potential of the now? After all, how many times have you seen the mighty oak wishing that it were a seedling again instead of reveling in the power and strength that it has now? Reassess what makes you sexy now, and go with that.

- **You're curious:** Curiosity is almost as sexy as confidence because it makes you inquisitive, thoughtful, empathetic, and forever youthful. Expressing genuine interest in others leads to their being interested in you in return. It also keeps you interested in learning something new every day, which is the very nexus of "sexy."

- **You understand how your body works:** It is difficult to change what you do not understand. Understanding the basics of how your body functions allows you to identify your current limitations more realistically because, while you may have limitless potential, you often have to start with the resources that are available now. For example, if your goal is to become more physically fit, and up to this point, you have primarily led a sedentary lifestyle, understanding that your body needs to be fueled differently to support muscle recovery and growth—your exercise increase needs to be gradual to allow for your heart and lung capacity to adapt—and that weight loss is not the ideal measurement of success, allows you to create goals that are consistent with where you are now. You can now appreciate that feeling more energetic and motivated are successful milestones. Use this success to fuel your next step, and so on and so on.

- **You know that you are meant to live your life out loud:** You have value. Accepting and acknowledging this simple fact allows you to know that you are good enough, talented enough, and smart enough, so you are not afraid to speak up, show up, and pursue your dreams. To quote Nelson Mandela, "There is no passion to be found playing small—in settling for a life that is less than the one you are capable of living."

- **You're here:** Seriously, the fact that you're curious, interested, and motivated to "get your sexy back" tells me one thing: you're already sexy. You just need a little information, confirmation, and validation to keep moving forward.

Sexercise:

A "Sexy Back" Activity

After each chapter, I'll feature a brief "Sexercise," which is an activity designed specifically to help you get your sexy back. For this first chapter, it's really simple—just fill in the blank below:

I feel sexiest when I am

_____.

If you find it difficult to complete this sentence, then take this opportunity to list the things you believe are preventing you from being healthy and sexy. This will help you identify the things you need to address to move forward. Doing so will help guide you as to what section of this book will provide you with the most insight to move forward from that space of inertia.

For example:

I would feel better about myself if

- I had more energy;

- I lost weight;

- I had someone to tell me I am sexy;

- I had more confidence;

- I could think more clearly;

- I slept better; and

- _____

_____

_____

_____.

Chapter 2: Healthy Brain

Peace of Mind, Prosperity of Thoughts, Purpose in Life

"Success is liking yourself, liking what you do, and liking how you

do it."

—*Maya Angelou*

When I think of the word *sexy*, it immediately brings to mind Maya Angelou's beautiful and moving poem "Phenomenal Woman." The poem's name may not immediately leap to your mind, but you've no doubt heard its powerful refrain:

> "I'm a woman
> Phenomenally.
>
> Phenomenal woman,
> That's me . . ."

My best friend gave this poem to me in a beautifully decorated frame several years ago as a birthday present. It has since become one of my most treasured possessions. I read and immerse myself in the words every time I need reminding of my strength, my ability, my femininity, and my sexiness. In that moment, I can feel that quiet confidence awaken and unfurl from deep within, bringing with it the peace of mind that comes from prosperity of thoughts, thus reminding me of my purpose: to be phenomenally myself at all times. Before too long, I can feel that lift in my chin and the sway in my hips, and no matter what I am wearing or how my hair looks, I feel sexy.

This poem and its wisdom, along with a lifetime of experiences, both personal and professional, have helped shape what "sexy" is to me. I have come to realize that sex appeal means strength with flexibility—so I won't break with the wind—confidence without the need for arrogance, and beauty that is reinforced by self-acceptance.

What is "sexy" to you? When you think of sexiness, what comes to your mind? Do you envision yourself vibrant, full of energy, and confident in your ability to look and feel your best? If not, then why not? What is holding you back from being able to see yourself as a sexy, vibrant person? Is it fatigue, mental fogginess, or less-than-optimal physical condition?

Maybe what's holding you back is a toxic environment, a job you hate, or a relationship (or relationships) that deplete rather than nourish your soul. It may even be a history of self-doubt that you have dragged with you from the past into each stage and interaction in your life. Perhaps your particular lifestyle habits, such as smoking, drinking, or overeating, rob rather than restore your vital energy.

As we began to explore in the first chapter, another important part of being sexy is your relationship with yourself. When was the last time you looked at yourself in the mirror and saw your limitless potential? When was the last time you saw that light in your eyes that illuminates your face or appreciated the curves of your hips and the pout of your lips? If the answer is, "I can't remember that far back," then it might be time to take action.

In this chapter, I'm going to teach you to harness the power of your brain to help you think and grow "sexy" and "healthy."

The Power of the Mind

It may surprise you to learn that the place to start your trip back to sexiness is with a healthy brain, so that you can engage the full power of the mind and begin to know and understand the true power of your sexiness. If you can feel it and think it, then you can start believing it. I have always thought that belief leads to confidence, confidence leads to acceptance, acceptance leads to love, and love leads to change. After all, most would agree that love is the impetus behind change. Most of us would take any action to support and protect the ones we love. Imagine if we felt that way about ourselves—what a powerful tool that would put into our hands.

Before we go any further, let's consider the principal question at hand: What is the mind? It is a simple enough question, but it is one that has confounded philosophers and scientists for a long time. While this debate can rage on for centuries, I have opted to choose a simple definition of the mind, one that helps me to exit the debate and move on to action. One definition that makes it easier for me to begin to grasp the power of the mind is the following: "The mind is the human consciousness that originates in the brain and is manifested, especially in thought, perception, emotion, will, memory, and imagination." Thank you, *Webster's Dictionary*!

In other words, we can use the power of our thoughts, our emotions, and even our imagination to influence the way we experience the world and, most importantly, the way we experience ourselves. It's critical to remember that sexiness starts from within. It starts in our belief that we are worthy of being healthy and of feeling attractive, sensual, and sexy. However, for others to believe it, we first have to believe it ourselves.

Many studies have shown, and continue to show, the powerful link between the mind and the body. For example, one of the more comprehensive meta-analysis studies published in the *Annals of Internal Medicine* reviewed over eighty studies centered around the effect of optimistic thinking (mind) on physical health (body).

This analysis is telling us that we can change the way we feel and our health by being conscious of what we think. These studies found that not only did optimistic thinkers subjectively feel better about themselves but they also fared better on objective criteria, such as mortality, immune system function and efficiency, cancer survival rates, and even pregnancy. So if the power of optimism can help you live longer, imagine harnessing that power to be the best version of you.

Now, let me take a brief moment to say what optimism means to me. Optimism, to me, is not thinking happy, unprompted thoughts all day long. As a human being, I am pretty sure that is an impossible feat. I prefer to think of optimism as hope fueled by action. Hope recognizes the challenges and constraints and obligations of life, but hope chooses to act on the things that can be changed, offers love to the person going through the challenge and knows that all things change. In doing so, hope positions itself to take the action necessary to help direct that change.

The Brain—Your Path to Mind over Matter

If what you think and feel about yourself is an important part of your health and well-being, then it stands to reason that the brain—the organ responsible for generating these thoughts and feelings—is of paramount importance. Not only does the brain stand guard over your feelings and thoughts but it also very much regulates almost all of the functions in your body. Functions that, when integrated with your thoughts and feelings, create the unique expression that is you.

Fun Facts about the Brain

The brain is fun, exciting, interesting, and—certainly by *Webster's* definition—sexy. After you peruse these fascinating facts about the brain, you will start to understand why a healthy brain is one of the first steps to a healthier, sexier you:

- The average human brain weighs about three pounds. Up to 60 percent of this is water weight. This makes the brain approximately 2 percent of the total body weight. Einstein's brain weighed 2.7 pounds, less than the average brain. So, as you can see, it is not the size of the brain but what you do with it.

- The brain has about one hundred billion neurons. A typical neuron has about one thousand to ten thousand synapses, or connections, to other nerve cells. Mind-blowing. One neuron can live for your entire lifetime. So, it is important to take care of them.

- The brain uses about 20 percent of the total body energy. That's right—it is 2 percent by weight but uses up 20 percent of the energy. There must be some pretty powerful work happening here. According to the University of Minnesota Medical School, two-thirds of that energy is used in helping the cells send signals and communicate, but a full one-third is used to maintain the health and well-being of the cell.

- The brain receives about 750 to 1,000 milliliters (equivalent to about three cans of soda) of oxygenated blood per minute. Loss of blood flow to the brain for about eight to ten seconds will result in a loss of consciousness, and brain cells will begin to die in about four to six minutes.

- Most interestingly, the Laboratory of Neuroimaging at the University of Southern California did a study that estimated that the average individual has about seventy thousand thoughts a day. These are seventy thousand opportunities to either boost your health, well-being, and sexiness or seventy thousand opportunities to do the opposite of that. Now you can begin to appreciate the importance of a healthy mind, healthy thoughts, and a healthy body.

While this information would provide an entertaining night playing Trivial Pursuit, I want you to think of it as information that helps you understand why it is necessary to take care of your brain's health. Change your thoughts; change your feelings. Change your feelings; change the way you experience the world. Changing the way you experience the world puts the control back into your hands. We need a healthy brain to begin to generate a healthy thought.

Nourish Your Brain

When your mind is functioning optimally, it is akin to that dream car you have always wanted, fresh off the assembly line. It is the ideal color and shape that perks your mood up just by looking at it. It accelerates like a dream, and when you apply the brake, it brings you to an effortlessly smooth stop. It handles like a dream and corners like it was made to be driven only by you. In my opinion, the brain is the conduit that helps the mind-body connection flow so seamlessly.

When we look at our definition of the mind—the human consciousness that originates in the brain and is manifested especially in thought, perception, emotion, will, memory, and imagination—we begin to see what an important tool this amazing organ is in helping us maintain our sense of general well-being.

We all know that "sexy" is about looking good, but it is also about feeling even better. That's because when you feel good, it not only shows on your face, skin, and body but it also inspires you to take action that helps you to look and feel even better. The better you feel, the more confident you are that you can do and be what you desire.

So how do we start on this path to feeling better? Do we wait until we like what we see in the mirror before we allow ourselves to feel good? Do we wait until we lose weight or have that surgery or clear up that acne?

Science and life experience tell us that waiting until we look better before we start to feel better actually may be delaying the very goal that we are trying to achieve. For example, berating ourselves about our weight may lead us to eat more high-sugar foods, to give up on exercise, and to feel more depressed due to the abundance of sugar and lack of exercise.

So one of the first steps to a healthy brain is to realize that toxicity to the brain comes in many forms, and the form that is constantly with us, but very seldom acknowledged, is our toxic thoughts and negative chatter. Remember, we have about seventy thousand thoughts a day. Imagine if 50 percent of those were self-critical thoughts. That would be thirty-five thousand negative thoughts a day. Wow, talk about a toxic environment! We simply have to stop talking poorly about ourselves *to* ourselves. I realize that this can be a lot more challenging to do in real life than it is to write about in a book, so I am going to get you started on the path with a step-by-step guidance tool.

Stopping negative chatter requires awareness of the negative self-talk and a conscious decision to change. Even with the decision made, realize that there might be neurochemical, structural, or electrical imbalances in the brain that may require additional help to overcome. For example, trauma can cause the brain to get stuck in a negative loop. When this occurs, professional help may be required to help us move forward.

Negative Chatter: Why It Matters

Brain cells that are constantly bathed in the toxic environment of negative self-talk cannot strive. You've heard the old adage that "you are what you eat." Well, new studies tell us that we are what we think. Many of us look at ourselves in the mirror, and our first thought is often a disparaging one: "I'm too fat. My stomach is too big. I hate my [fill in the blank]." Or we might say, "If only I had a more toned butt or leaner thighs, then I would love myself more—and others would love me as well." Stop and ask yourself whose thoughts are you repeating? Are they your thoughts, or are they fueled by a critical parent from the past making comments about your weight or a judgmental spouse's seemingly offhand comments about something you are wearing? At this point, these thoughts may have been with you for so long and have integrated themselves so deeply into your neurochemistry that it is impossible to identify their origin.

According to the Mayo Clinic, thinking positively—or having an optimistic attitude—lowers rates of depression, increases life spans, and improves the ability to handle stress, thereby improving physical and emotional well-being.

Conversely, bathing your brain in toxic thoughts that chronically elevate stress hormones can lead to the death of brain cells, poor memory, poor sleep quality, and mood disorders—most commonly anxiety or depression. One study showed that optimism—or positive thoughts—actually increased the levels of BDNF (brain-derived neurotropic factor), a compound found in the brain whose job it is to protect and nourish brain cells. Exercise has also been shown to increase the levels of this amazing substance.

Normal levels of BDNF are also associated with a decreased risk of depression and a better response to antidepressant treatment and medication. To top it all off, studies show that higher levels of

BDNF have been associated with a decreased risk of Alzheimer's disease and dementia.

Do you still doubt the power of positive thinking? Then I give you the golf-putting experiment published in the *Journal of Cognitive Research*. College students were divided into three groups for this groundbreaking study. The first group was asked to visualize its putt going into the hole, the second group was allowed to putt without instructions, and the last group was asked to imagine the ball barely missing the hole.

Guess which group displayed better motor skill accuracy by getting the ball in the hole more often? You guessed it: the positive visualization group. Who did the worst? Once again, I'm sure you figured it out—the negative visualization group.

So what can you do if you feel that your life and your feelings are being controlled by a sea of negativity? Well, according to Dr. David Burns, a prominent researcher and psychiatrist at Stanford University in California, you must first identify the thought causing you distress, and replace it with a positive thought that you believe more.

Notice, he didn't say replace negative thoughts with random positive thoughts. Instead, he urges us to isolate one negative thought and replace it with a conceivable, believable positive thought. This might be the reason so many of us are coming up short when we try to employ the power of positive thinking.

Dr. Burns' years of research and treating patients have shown that the positive thoughts with the most impact are those the individual believes to be 100 percent true and, also, happen to make the original negative thought untrue.

In fact, this is one of the tools used in a very successful form of therapy called cognitive behavioral therapy (CBT), which is used to treat mood disorders such as anxiety and even depression. This form of therapy has been shown in many studies to be just as effective as—and in some cases, more effective—than medication. Even when medication was used, the effectiveness was enhanced when it was combined with CBT.

Learning to replace negative thoughts with positive ones, and understanding the importance behind quieting your negative thoughts, is the first step toward thinking your way to "sexy." But there is more to do, and we've only just begun.

Power Your Brain with Healthy Nutrients, Sleep, Exercise, and Hydration

A healthy brain requires good nutrients, adequate sleep, lots of hydration, nurturing relationships, a healthy environment, a tangible stress-management strategy, balanced brain waves, encouraging thoughts, exercise, and stimulation. Engaging in daily learning activities and challenges turns the brain's potential energy into kinetic energy, thus keeping it well tuned. A brain that is at optimal capacity is the foundation of any intervention, whether it is therapy, medication, or lifestyle intervention.

Nutrients and the Brain

We've heard the saying, "You are what you eat." Well, this is particularly true when it comes to the brain. As you recall, the brain is made of billions of neurons, and an estimated 60 percent of brain matter is composed of fat and approximately 70 percent water by weight. It is only 2 percent of the body's weight, but it uses up over 20 percent of our daily energy consumption. It is estimated that two-thirds of the brain's energy is channeled toward active processes while a full one-third goes toward keeping the brain ready for action at all times. This high energy consumption leads to a high production of free radicals, leaving the brain open to the effects of oxidative stress. Thus, eating for brain health requires not only foods that provide fuel for the brain but also foods that provide high antioxidant value, which offers protection to the billions of cells that make up the brain.

For example, eating foods that are high in sugar or highly processed foods that contain trans fats has been shown to create inflammation in the brain and simply does not provide adequate nutrients for top-notch brain function. So it is a double whammy—increased oxidation without proper nutrients. Conversely, omega-3 fatty acids have been shown to improve communication between neurons, to decrease anxiety, to improve depression, and to decrease inflammation in the brain. Fats help form the membranes around the cells, as well as provide insulation and protection for the axons of the neurons or nerve cells. This fatty layer of protection is called the myelin sheath. Damage to this layer can lead to neurodegenerative conditions such as multiple sclerosis.

If omega-3 fats are replaced by trans fats—most frequently found in fast and processed foods—in and around the brain cells, energy production goes down, oxidative stress increases, and brain cells cannot communicate well with each other. It is akin to putting used oil in your car or cooking with oil that has previously been superheated. Imagine the look of burnt oil, brown and smoking— that is a good example of your brain on trans fats. You can see how a sludgy brain can find it difficult to think clearly.

Other important nutrients that support healthy brain function include the B vitamins, such as folic acid, niacin, vitamin B6, and vitamin B12. These B vitamins help keep nerve cells healthy and keep levels of neurotransmitters normal, which are special chemicals in the brain and body used for cell-to-cell communication. These neurotransmitters play an important role in moods, energy, and our ability to enjoy the things life has to offer.

A well-balanced supply of amino acids from healthy protein sources is also needed for neurotransmitters in the brain to process emotions, to maintain focus, to enhance learning, and to generate a sense of well-being and calm in the midst of chaos. An example of this is the amino acid tryptophan used in making the neurotransmitter serotonin. Part of serotonin's function is to help us maintain a balanced mood. Interestingly, serotonin is also converted into melatonin in the brain, and we have come to realize the important role that melatonin plays in our sleep cycle. Studies suggest that melatonin may also play a role in fortifying our immune system to decrease our risk of certain cancers.

Not to be left out of the brain health foray, magnesium has been shown in studies to be a key player in maintaining healthy brain function. Research continues to elucidate magnesium's role in brain health—from helping us maintain a sense of calm to enhancing memory functions, thus making it easier for us to adjust our thought patterns.

Now that we have these nutrients hard at work to help keep us happy, healthy, and sexy, a diet high in antioxidants is needed to help protect the brain from the ravages of damaging free radicals that are produced on a daily basis during the production of neurotransmitters and other essential neurochemical reactions. Remember, the brain accounts for up to 20 percent of the energy utilized by the body. As you can imagine, this amount of metabolism can lead to the production of significant waste products that would need to be neutralized. In fact, some scientists now believe that many neurodegenerative diseases, such as Parkinson's disease, are fueled by excessive oxidative stress. Now, imagine all these nutrients working in harmony. It would be like a happy cocktail for your brain. So, as you can see, a healthy, balanced diet is an integral part of thinking and being sexy.

Sleep: Beyond Closing Your Eyes

What is sleep? According to *Merriam-Webster's Dictionary*, "Sleep is the natural periodic suspension of consciousness during which the powers of the body are restored." This description tells us that sleep is the body's and the brain's rest and renewal cycle and, therefore, is a critical component of good health. While bodily functions, such as respiration, heart rate, and blood pressure are lowered during the sleep cycle, sleep is by no means a passive process. The benefits of sleep can range from speeding up recovery from the common cold to playing a significant role in helping us form and retain memories.

How Does Sleep Work?

Sleep, while it may appear to be a serene process, is quite a complex physiological dance between neurotransmitters, genetics, circadian rhythm, and hormones. I understand that you are not reading this book to obtain a biology degree, so I promise to keep it simple.

Stages of Sleep

Sleep happens in two general stages: REM (rapid eye movement) and NREM (nonrapid eye movement). NREM sleep is about 80 percent of the sleep cycle. The American Academy of Sleep has recommended that NREM sleep be divided into three stages based on brain wave patterns.

N1 Sleep: This is the transition from wakefulness to sleep, often referred to as light sleep. If you have ever experienced a sense of falling followed by a sudden muscle jerk, you most likely were in this stage of sleep. This is known as hypnic myoclonia.

N2 Sleep: This is the "real deal" sleep. We spend about 40 percent to 50 percent of NREM sleep in this stage.

N3 Sleep: This is slow brain wave sleep, or deep sleep. About 20 percent is spent in this stage of sleep.

REM Sleep

As the name suggests, rapid eye movement is characteristic of this stage of sleep. Interestingly, in this stage of sleep, the rest of the voluntary muscles in the body are inactive. Heart rate, respirations, and blood pressure increase during this phase of sleep. The brain wave pattern seen in REM is fast and low voltage, similar to wave patterns that are seen in the wake cycle. REM sleep is also where dreaming occurs. We spend about 20 to 25 percent of the time in this stage of sleep.

In general, we spend more time in NREM earlier in the night and more time in REM in the latter half of the full sleep cycle. We enter our first REM sleep about seventy to ninety minutes after we fall asleep. Going through the entire sleep cycle takes about 90 to 110 minutes. Then, the cycles repeat, though not necessarily in order.

Interference to any one of these stages could cause issues and sleep disorders. For example, certain antidepressants can suppress REM sleep. Alcohol may make it easier to enter into the light sleep cycle but decreases REM and restorative deep sleep, therefore leaving you feeling unrefreshed. Remember, during the light sleep cycle, we can be aroused very easily. Heavy smoking can create a similar disturbance to alcohol-induced sleep. Sleep studies can help us identify the stage at which sleep interruption occurs, as treatment may differ depending on the stage.

Sleep Disorders

It is estimated that we spend approximately one-third of our lives sleeping. If we are required to sleep for 33 percent of our lives to function optimally, it must be important. Anyone who has ever suffered from a sleep disorder can attest to the far-reaching effects of disruption of the natural sleep cycle. Statistics tells us that at least 80 percent of people suffer from transient insomnia (insomnia lasting less than two weeks). This means that at least 80 percent of the population will have times when they have difficulty falling or staying asleep. As the name implies, this oftentimes resolves spontaneously or with some adjustments in lifestyle or behavioral treatment. It is also estimated that 15 percent of the population suffers from chronic insomnia. Insomnia is just one expression of sleep disorders. While there are currently over ninety defined sleep disorders, sleep disorders can be categorized into three basic groups:

- Those causing trouble falling asleep or staying asleep (also referred to as insomnia)
- Those causing daytime sleepiness as the primary complaint
- Those associated with disruptive behavior during sleep

Treatment for sleep disorders is based on the type of sleep disorder, the stage of sleep that it impacts, and the dysfunction it produces. Sometimes, treating one sleep disorder can significantly impact another part of the sleep cycle, thereby potentially creating other concerns. For example, short-term sleep disorders are often prescribed a sedative to help induce sleep. Benzodiazepines are a class of medications that are often used to treat insomnia. This class of medication is known to suppress REM sleep. REM sleep plays an important role in pulling together memory and learning. It therefore follows that the use of these medications could potentially impact daytime memory and performance. In fact, long-term use of this class of medication has been linked to an increased risk of dementia in the elderly. So, if you suffer from chronic sleep deprivation, it is important to not only determine what is causing the disruption but also what part of the cycle is being affected so that treatment can be targeted to reduce potential unwanted issues.

Circadian Rhythm and Sleep

Circadian rhythms are biological changes that occur in roughly twenty-four-hour cycles that are triggered primarily by light. Did you know that most people's natural clock runs on twenty-five-hour cycles? Circadian rhythm helps to determine when we go to sleep and when we wake up and also controls many of the hormonal functions of the body. Our circadian rhythm is controlled by a "master clock" in the brain. This master clock is made up of two groups—located on both sides of the brain—of about twenty thousand neurons called the suprachiasmatic nuclei located in the hypothalamus. The hypothalamus is located strategically above where the optic nerves (responsible for vision) cross. This location allows the suprachiasmatic nucleus to access information about incoming light. Incoming light enters the eye, hits the retina in the back of the eye, and then this information is transmitted to the SCN. Light then is able to turn on and off the genes that control the body's internal clocks via this direct connection to the brain. Imagine—light can have an impact on turning on and off our genes.

There are many things besides light that can impact our circadian rhythm. For example, traveling across time zones, certain medications, late-night shift work, pregnancy, and certain diseases, such as Alzheimer's, can cause a disruption in this cycle. I am sure that many of us have experienced what it feels like to have our circadian rhythm thrown off course when we travel across time zones, such as traveling from California to Florida. Our sleep gets disrupted, we may feel fatigued, or our bowel function may be impaired by this seemingly minor change in time. This is commonly referred to as jet lag, and it takes a few days for the body to adjust to the new time zone.

The influence of the body's circadian rhythm extends well beyond our sleep/wake cycle. Studies show that a disruption of the circadian rhythm can contribute to diseases such as diabetes, seasonal affective disorder, depression, and other mood disorders. Some studies, such as those done in night-shift workers, even show a link between a desynchronized circadian rhythm and an increased risk of certain cancers. Since the circadian rhythm influences biological factors, such as hormonal release and body temperature, one can see how it is possible for a disruption in these processes to lead to pathological conditions.

Genes and the Circadian Rhythm

Do genes play a role in determining how much sleep we need to function at our best or how well we handle a disruption in our circadian rhythm? Researchers have found that there are genes that determine how circadian rhythm works. This may help to explain why some individuals seem to do well on just six hours of sleep, while others require a full eight hours in order to function optimally. Research conducted at the University of California, San Francisco, found that individuals with a mutation in a gene called DEC2 can function normally with just six hours of sleep. This is without a power nap during the day. Keep in mind that these genetic mutations do not appear to be a common occurrence. They are estimated to occur in one in every sixty families. Most individuals who sleep for only six hours a night exhibit signs and symptoms of sleep deprivation.

Treating Circadian Disorders

How do you get your circadian rhythm back on track? If it is caused by medication, then speak to your doctor about options. Circadian-rhythm disruption is oftentimes successfully treated with behavioral-modification therapies:

Chronotherapy: This is a fancy name for a treatment that focuses on gradually adjusting your bedtime until you get to the desired bedtime. For example, if you find yourself going to bed at 3:00 a.m. nightly and your desired bedtime is 11:00 p.m., gradually adjust your bedtime by an hour or so until you get to bed at 11:00 p.m. Once there, be consistent.

Bright-light therapy: Exposure to bright light at a specified intensity and duration can help certain individuals who suffer from a circadian-rhythm disruption.

Improving sleep hygiene: This simply means to develop habits that promote sleep and to do away with habits that keep you awake.

- Avoid bright-light exposure at bedtime. That includes removing television, computers, and telephones from your sleep environment.
- Keep the room dark and quiet. Pay attention to the room temperature.
- Eliminate sleep disruptors, such as caffeine, cigarettes, and alcohol, especially at night. Some individuals are so

sensitive to caffeine that ingesting it any later than noon can lead to a night of tossing and turning.

- Avoid vigorous exercise at least three hours prior to bed.
- Avoid taking long naps during the day. Twenty-minute naps can be a good way to invigorate your afternoon, but sleeping for too long during the day can disrupt your sleep pattern at night.

Neurotransmitters and Sleep

Numerous neurotransmitters and neuropeptides play important roles in maintaining your circadian rhythm. Scientists are discovering new ones every day. Below is a brief list of some of the neurotransmitters that can impact our sleep.

Orexin: Orexin is a neuropeptide produced in the hypothalamus that contributes to the wakefulness part of the cycle. In fact, it is thought that a deficiency in orexin contributes to narcolepsy. Excessive orexin production can contribute to sleep disorders. The newest sleep aid Belsomra works by inhibiting the actions of this neurotransmitter.

Acetylcholine: Acetylcholine levels differ depending on what stage of sleep you are in. Levels are high in REM sleep and lower in the slow-wave phase of sleep. Light seems to increase the amount of acetylcholine in the SCN.

Norepinephrine: Believe it or not, this stimulatory neurotransmitter plays a role in stimulating the pineal gland to manufacture the sleep hormone melatonin. It helps with the conversion of the amino acid tryptophan into melatonin.

Cortistatin: Cortistatin is a newly discovered neuropeptide that plays a role in inducing the slow-wave phase of sleep. It is thought to antagonize the stimulatory effect of the activity of acetylcholine, thus decreasing neuronal activity.

Hormones and Sleep: How Do Hormones Impact the Circadian Rhythm?

Hormones are chemical substances produced by different cells in the body and are transported to distant sites to regulate function elsewhere in the body. Many of these hormones have been shown to play a significant role in sleep. Below is a brief description of some of the key hormones that we know so far:

Melatonin: As mentioned above, the pair of nuclei called the suprachiasmatic nuclei (SCN) controls the body's internal clock. These nuclei are located above where the optic nerves cross and, therefore, are in the ideal position to receive information about ambient light. Information from the SCN is then passed on to the pineal gland through a series of complicated neurological pathways. The pineal gland is then stimulated to make and secrete melatonin, one of our primary sleep hormones. As we get older, our pineal gland is prone to calcification, and this causes a reduction in the production of melatonin. It is theorized that this could be one of the reasons older individuals suffer from more sleep disturbances. Interestingly, some initial research links increased calcification of the pineal gland to movement disorders, such as tardive dyskinesia and Tourette's.

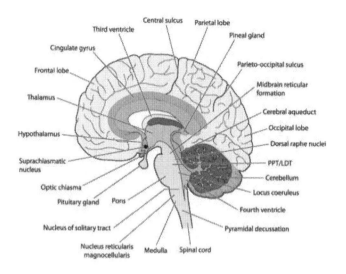

Figure 2.1

Studies suggest that melatonin's role in the body extends well beyond getting a good night's sleep. For example, melatonin is thought to play a role in regulating the normal growth of cells. Melatonin in the elderly seems to improve mild cognitive impairment. This is in contrast to studies that suggest that the use of benzodiazepines, used commonly to treat sleep disorders, can actually increase the risk of cognitive impairment.

Other hormones: The pattern of secretion of almost all hormones influences the circadian rhythm and the sleep cycle. For example, testosterone levels are highest in the morning for men.

Cortisol, one of our primary stress hormones, has a circadian rhythm that peaks in the morning and is at its lowest at night. We know that the secretion of cortisol is controlled by the HPA axis (hypothalamic-pituitary-adrenal axis). What has been recently discovered is that the SCN master clock in the hypothalamus seems to have a direct connection to the adrenal glands via the sympathetic nervous system. This then would put the SCN with direct influence over the function of the adrenal glands and, thus, the production of cortisol. As you can imagine, desynchronization of these hormonal levels can wreak havoc on the body and your health.

While this is in no way an exhaustive list of the neurochemicals involved in sleep and circadian-rhythm regulation, I hope it gives you some idea of how much energy and resources the body puts into ensuring that you get a good night's sleep. It should also give you an appreciation of the complexity of potential causes of sleep disorders, and why oftentimes it may take a multimodal approach to get you back to that restorative sleep that seems so elusive.

Hydration

What does hydration have to do with it? As mentioned earlier, the brain is estimated to be 70 percent water by weight. Research suggests that dehydration can actually cause brain tissue to shrink. A functional MRI study published in *Human Brain Mapping* in 2011 revealed that decrease in hydration causes the brain to use much more energy and many more resources to accomplish a routine cognitive task. Imagine the brain trying to function in a constant state of dehydration and expending excessive amounts of energy to accomplish a routine task. In my opinion, this can potentially lead to the production of an excessive amount of damaging oxidative stress from the increased metabolism, and as mentioned earlier, many neurological dysfunctions are now being linked to increased free radical damage to the brain's neurons.

Studies also suggest that your perception of pain will be greater when you are dehydrated. Research also suggests that a 2 percent decrease in hydration status can negatively impact immediate memory skills, impair psychomotor function, contribute to lower mood, and even cause us to feel physical discomfort, such as a headache. So while you may still remember how to put one foot in front of the other, it will certainly seem more of a challenge than it should, and you certainly won't feel good about it.

Who can feel sexy when it is a struggle to think and walk straight? Athletes have known this secret for years; now, you too can take advantage of this information. And it's so easy to remedy this situation—by just drinking more.

Exercise

Why do you exercise? The majority of Americans will probably say that they use exercise to "lose or maintain weight." Yet, studies tell us that people who use weight loss as motivation to exercise actually exercise less frequently than those who use exercise as a wellness tool. When you use exercise as a wellness tool, oftentimes, you can appreciate the immediate benefits such as increased energy, clearer thinking, and improved moods. You can see and feel the benefits. This motivates you to continue and build on your routine. When your sole measurement of success is dependent on a number on a scale decreasing at a particular rate, then it is easier for the frustration to build when that number remains stagnant or even increases. You can very quickly become discouraged and start feeling that all of your efforts are for naught. Why continue an action if you are not getting results? Maybe the better question is, are you using the right tools to measure your success?

Studies show that exercise improves moods, sometimes just as well as an antidepressant drug. Exercise increases the brain's protective BDNF, thus helping us to maintain a positive mood. Exercise—again, most likely through BDNF—has been shown to promote neurogenesis, or the growth of new, healthier nerve cells. In fact, research done at the University of British Columbia showed that regular aerobic exercise increases the size of the hippocampus, a structure in the brain that plays an important role in memory and learning. This is important, especially when it is estimated that in the year 2050, approximately 115 million people worldwide will be diagnosed with dementia in some form.

Exercise seems to affect brain and body health via multiple mechanisms. There are very few, if any, pharmaceuticals that can make that claim. This simple act of keeping the body in motion improves insulin sensitivity, decreases inflammation, decreases anxiety, and improves depression, all of which contribute to a happier, healthier brain. Yes, exercise can give you the toned look you desire, but in my opinion, a healthy, strong mind is the cornerstone to true sexiness.

A Healthy Dose of Nature a Day Helps to Keep Depression Away

Have you ever noticed that being outside in nature seems to have the ability to enhance your moods? Whether you have ever been hypnotized by the ebb and flow of the ocean waves or drawn into the dance of the trees as the wind rustles through their leaves and branches, or you have ever simply turned your face up to the sun to feel the warmth caress your cheek, you have been influenced by the power of nature. You find yourself releasing the tension of the day, your chaotic thoughts seem to recede to some quiet corner of your mind, and, as the feeling of peace slowly surrounds you, you find yourself able to take long, deep breaths as if breathing in the very essence of life. That is the symbiotic relationship we have with nature and our environment. When nature thrives, we thrive.

What we have known intuitively for generations, studies now support—even the simulation of nature can have a significant positive impact on our mental and physical well-being. In 2010, researchers from multiple universities coauthored a study on the "Vitalizing Effects of Nature," which was published in the *Journal of Environmental Psychology*. The authors wanted to determine the impact of nature on energy, independent of physical activity. They also wanted to answer the burning question could visualization of nature be just as energizing as physically being in nature? The researchers designed five different experiments involving 537 college students. All five scenarios came to a similar conclusion: Mother Nature, real or imagined, had a significant impact in boosting energy levels and moods in as little as twenty minutes a day. Take-away point: taking a few minutes a day to immerse yourself with the sound of water as it gently flows downstream, as the wind gently rustles through the leaves, while you imagine being in your favorite spot in nature, may be just the shot of energy you need to keep your day on track.

Your Brain on Friendship

Do you want to think, feel, and grow sexier? Then surround yourself with nourishing friendships and a cooperative environment. Study after study tells us that individuals with strong social networks and bonds of friendships live longer, are happier, and feel better about themselves.

People with strong social ties handle stress better. It is postulated that some of the biochemistry behind this fact may involve the bonding hormone oxytocin. This is the same hormone that is secreted during breastfeeding and labor, presumably to facilitate mom-and-baby bonding.

Fortunately for us, this is not the only time that this chemical is secreted. This hormone also helps us feel closer to each other. In fact, studies show that higher oxytocin levels are associated with increased levels of trust, happiness, and a sense of well-being.

Individuals with close friendships secrete more oxytocin and, therefore, may experience a greater sense of happiness.

When we are happier, our thoughts are more optimistic. When our thoughts are more optimistic, our bodies generate less inflammation and stress hormones. When our bodies generate less inflammation and stress hormones, our risk for chronic diseases decreases, we have more energy, we eat better, we exercise more, and we are healthier. In other words, we are sexier!

But hold on, just when you thought the story of oxytocin was complete, there is another wrinkle to consider. It appears that oxytocin, in certain cases, can actually generate or worsen anxiety symptoms. A study published in the journal *Biological Psychiatry* seems to suggest that oxytocin may just intensify the effects of social interaction when it is present in a particular part of the brain. For example, if you are feeling anxious being in a setting with unfamiliar people at a party, then the presence of oxytocin can magnify this feeling, thus, perhaps, potentially worsening symptoms of social anxiety. If, however, you are with family and friends that you adore, then the presence of oxytocin can enhance that feeling of being loved and cherished. Keep in mind that this study was done on rats and more study is needed to clarify this occurrence in humans.

As far as friendships go, studies are suggesting that it may be more important for women to have healthy friendships in order to combat stress and its negative impact. Numerous studies have shown that negative emotions have a stronger impact on a woman's emotional brain than on a man's emotional brain. In short, women respond more strongly to negative emotions. This may again lead back to the above study. It seems that the two areas of the brain that seem to respond strongly to oxytocin, the bed nucleus of the stria terminalis (BNST), which controls anxiety, and the nucleus accumbens, which plays a role in reward and motivation, are more active in female brains. Of course, this statement raises a "but why?" The truth is we don't know the specifics right now. We are just beginning to explore and understand the complexities of the male and female brains.

In an attempt to further that understanding, Stanford University researchers looked at the brains of twelve men and twelve women using functional MRI studies. The study involved evaluating the brain of these individuals while they were looking at neutral and negative emotionally charged images. They evaluated the areas of the brain activated when participants viewed photos. They also tested the participants' memories three weeks after the initial exposure to measure recall of the images. Researchers discovered that women remembered the negative, emotionally charged images in more detail than their male counterparts. In other words, if an event is associated with a negative emotional connotation, the female brain records and remembers it in great detail. It is thought that this is one of the possible reasons that women are more susceptible to emotional disorders, such as depression and anxiety. They also noted that the female brain and the male brain utilized different neural pathways with different intensity. The male circuitry involved more of the right amygdala, while the female circuitry depended more on the left amygdala.

The exact opposite was noted to be true for a man's brain. A man's emotional brain will pay more attention to positive emotions than to negative emotions. It seems that when men experience positive emotions, the left amygdala is more activated. Remember, women exposed to negative emotions show higher activity in the left amygdala, while men show higher activity in the right amygdala. The take-home point is that men and women process emotional stimuli differently, and we are just beginning to scratch the surface.

The good news is that during stress events, women who bond with other women seem to produce more oxytocin, or the "love" hormone that encourages the "tend and befriend" response. According to a study done at the University of California, Los Angeles, women bonding with other women produced higher oxytocin levels, and this generated a greater sense of calm. As mentioned previously, oxytocin works best as a calming hormone when it is recruited during a positive emotional-bonding experience. So it seems that a "girls' night out" is actually an important part of managing stress and helping you get your "sexy" back.

In men, oxytocin did not seem to produce that same degree of calming during a bonding experience. It is postulated that testosterone can possibly interfere with the calming effects of oxytocin. Also, men might already have the built-in protection of their brain being able to prioritize positive experiences over negative experiences, so they may not be as reliant on oxytocin to help mediate the stress response.

Plan of Action

So what is the plan? How much should you sleep? What should you eat? How much should you drink? How frequently should you exercise? First, let's get rid of the word *should*. If we are honest with ourselves, we find that this word comes with a sense of built-in resistance. We may feel that we are constantly being told what we should do, how we should be, and what we should wear for our age, our status, our jobs, and so forth. Oftentimes, we take away from these interactions that somehow, in some way, we are not measuring up or we are not enough.

Life experience tells us that starting at, "I am not enough," is not an effective beginning if we want to create a new pattern. Perhaps the question that we can ask is, "What am I willing and able to do right now?" You are enough to start making small changes to accomplish what you want to do. You are enough to start feeling good about the core you. You are enough to realize that you are not broken. You are enough, period! Keep in mind that you don't have to wake up the next day with an entirely new set of habits, patterns, and lifestyle modifications. In other words, you can make changes one tiny step at a time. The goal is consistency, not great quantity, in short spurts. Start with one area of your life that you feel willing and able to begin changing.

How Much Sleep Do You Need?

Let's refresh. Lack of sleep has been shown to impair judgment and focus; to increase inflammation; to set us up for obesity, hypertension, and diabetes; and possibly, increase our risk of certain cancers. Functional MRI studies confirm that lack of sleep negatively impacts the higher functioning parts of our brains, and this actually leads to our making poor food choices, such as consuming high-sugar foods. Interference with the higher functioning areas of the brain, such as the medial prefrontal cortex (MPFC), can also affect the impact this area has on modulating the emotional part of our brain, the amygdala. This can leave us at risk for a more amplified response to negative emotional stimuli. To simplify, when we are working with a sleep deficit, we are more likely to "lose it" when faced with situations that are not ideal.

As sleep deprivation continues, poor decision making can be compounded. For example, lack of sleep can induce fatigue; fatigue then discourages exercise; lack of exercise leads to a decrease in muscle mass, which puts us at an increased risk of falling, increasing the risk of insulin resistance, and making us look and feel weak and frail. Put all these things together, and you may have a recipe for becoming fat, forgetful, frumpy, foggy, and fatigued—definitely not sexy.

So how much sleep is required to offset this vicious cycle? To answer this question, I defer to the National Sleep Foundation, which gathered eighteen experts in their respective fields to review over three hundred research articles and to come to a general consensus. As one would expect, individual needs will vary, but most of us will feel best in and around the recommended ranges listed below. To fine-tune the recommendations for you, you will need to pay attention to how you feel and function with even a slight modification in your sleep patterns. For example, do you feel refreshed and ready to face the day after seven hours of sleep or eight hours of sleep? Do you need a pot of espresso the next day to get you from point A to point B? Paying attention to how you feel and function the next day can help to alert you to potential sleep deprivation.

Below are the recommendations put forth by the National Sleep Foundation:

- **Newborns (zero to three months):** Sleep range has been narrowed to fourteen to seventeen hours each day (previously it was twelve to eighteen).

- **Infants (four to eleven months)**: Sleep range has been widened two hours to twelve to fifteen hours (previously it was fourteen to fifteen).

- **Toddlers (one to two years)**: Sleep range has been widened by one hour to eleven to fourteen hours (previously it was twelve to fourteen).

- **Preschoolers (three to five)**: Sleep range has been widened by one hour to ten to thirteen hours (previously it was eleven to thirteen).

- **School-age children (six to thirteen)**: Sleep range has been widened by one hour to nine to eleven hours (previously it was ten to eleven).

- **Teenagers (fourteen to seventeen)**: Sleep range has been widened by one hour to eight to ten hours (previously it was 8.5 to 9.5).

- **Younger adults (eighteen to twenty-five)**: Sleep range is seven to nine hours (new age category).

- **Adults (twenty-six to sixty-four)**: Sleep range did not change and remains seven to nine hours.

- **Older adults (sixty-five and older)**: Sleep range is seven to eight hours (new age category).

What Is the Prescription for Exercise?

Is there a magical number of minutes per week that confers all the benefits that exercise has to offer? Is exercise a "go big, or go home" phenomenon? According to the National Institute of Health, just thirty minutes a day, five days a week of moderate exercise can reduce the risk of dying by 27 percent. If thirty minutes sounds like a lot, then increase the intensity of the exercise, and you can exercise for just twenty minutes a day, three or more days a week, decreasing the risk of dying further by 32 percent. Vigorous exercise sounds daunting? Not to worry—a more recent study, published in the *Lancet* in 2011, looked at over four hundred thousand people over a twelve-year period and found that fifteen minutes a day of moderate exercise (brisk walking), six days a week, confers a very similar increase in longevity. My stance is that everyone has to start somewhere. So if five minutes is what you can do today, then do that. Something trumps nothing every time.

For brain health in particular, aerobic exercise, or exercise that gets the heart rate pumping, was more beneficial in making positive changes in the brain. Even better news, it takes as little as six months for those important areas in the brain to start increasing in volume. More important is that you will start feeling better and thinking more clearly well before then.

Protect the Brain: Antioxidants to the Rescue

Can certain nutrients help keep our brains healthy and, perhaps, decrease our risk of disorders such as Parkinson's and Alzheimer's? Studies suggest that this indeed could be the case. For example, it is thought that reactive oxygen species (free radicals) contribute to the development of many neurological disorders, such as Parkinson's and Alzheimer's. Research published in the *Journal of Neurochemistry* in 2009 showed that dopaminergic cells that have lower glutathione levels (one of the body's best antioxidants) are more susceptible to free-radical damage than cells with higher levels of glutathione. This theory would suggest that an overproduction of free radicals produced during normal functioning of the brain can potentially damage the neurons or brain cells enough to produce symptoms of neurological damage present in the aforementioned disorders. The immediate follow-up question is- can we supply enough antioxidants to potentially protect our brain cells from damage? Of course, as you have probably guessed, there is always much more to the story, but until we have the entire story, there are several studies that give us hope for the future.

Curcumin

Curcumin is derived from the turmeric root, a popular spice used in many East Indian and Caribbean cuisines. Studies tell us that this may be one of Mother Nature's best gifts to us, especially when it comes to the brain. Remember when I mentioned that glutathione was one of the body's best antioxidants that seemed to offer significant protection to brain cells? Well, research shows that curcumin has the ability to increase the production of glutathione in the brain, thus, perhaps, offering more protection to the brain. The news may be even better than this! Numerous animal studies show that through a variety of other mechanisms, curcumin administered prior to an ischemic event to the brain or stroke decreased the amount of damage caused by the stroke and improved recovery from the neurological deficits. In other words, the lasting effects of the stroke were much less.

The news gets better! Researchers at the medical school at UCLA made a startling discovery: combining vitamin D and curcumin helped to clear out the toxic substance that builds up during Alzheimer's disease called amyloid beta. It seems that vitamin D helps improve the clearance ability of one form of the body's scavengers called macrophages, and curcumin improved the function of another class of macrophage, thus packing a one-two punch that can, hopefully, be useful in treating this insidious, soul-stealing disease in the future.

N-Acetylcysteine

Many researchers believe glutathione is the major antioxidant in the brain that helps clear out the debris and damage created during normal function of the brain on a daily basis. One research study by Jeremy W. Gawryluk, published in the February 1, 2011 issue of *International Journal of Neuropsychopharmacology*, did an evaluation to compare the brains of individuals with major psychiatric disorders to the brains of individuals without a psychiatric diagnosis at the time of death. They found that the brains of the individuals with diagnoses, such as major depressive disorder and bipolar disorder had significantly lower levels of glutathione compared to the brains of the individuals who did not carry a psychiatric diagnosis.

Now, it would be ideal if replenishing glutathione would improve symptoms of these disorders. There are some small studies that suggest that in certain individuals that may be the case. P. V. Magalhães and others, in a study published in the *Journal of Affective Disorders* in March 2011, divided fourteen patients diagnosed with bipolar depression into two groups. The first group was assigned to receive a placebo and the second group to receive N-acetylcysteine. Neither the researcher nor the patient knew which one was being given. They followed the patients for twenty-four weeks. They reported that six of the seven in the N-acetylcysteine group had complete remission of depressive and manic symptoms, compared to only two in the placebo group. N-acetylcysteine is thought to work by enhancing the body's production of glutathione. Now, clearly, larger studies are needed, but who would be willing to invest in a study without much chance of significant financial return?

Alpha-Lipoic Acid

Alpha-lipoic acid is another antioxidant used ubiquitously in the body to help fight free radical damage. This remarkable compound that occurs naturally in the body has also been shown to support many other functions as well. For example, it is required as a cofactor in the mitochondria to help the body convert glucose into usable energy. As you may already know, the mitochondria are tiny energy-producing factories present inside the majority of cells in the body. The higher the amount of energy required by the cell, the more mitochondria it contains. If you recall, the brain uses 20 percent of the body's metabolic requirement. You can imagine the amount of energy it takes to keep this engine running smoothly. If alpha-lipoic acid is an essential part of this energy production, you can now get the sense of its importance.

Alpha-lipoic acid doesn't stop there—as part of the team responsible for keeping this engine running smoothly, it seems to also have the ability to clean up after itself. Simply stated, it has the ability to neutralize free radicals and increase the production of glutathione, one of the major antioxidants in the body. In addition, in the lab, alpha-lipoic acid has been shown to decrease inflammation by limiting the production of inflammatory substances, such as tumor necrosis factor. This cytokine is implicated in many chronic illnesses and autoimmune disorders, as well as mood disorders. Alpha-lipoic acid has one more trick up its sleeve when it comes to protecting the brain from potential harm—it seems to have the ability to increase the production of the neurotransmitter acetylcholine. This is important because acetylcholine is one of the neurotransmitters that plays a significant role in our memory functioning the way that it should. In fact, many of the pharmaceuticals targeted to treat Alzheimer's disease work by increasing the available acetylcholine levels.

The big question is, of course, does this translate into real-life protection? Two published studies looked at individuals with mild dementia versus individuals with moderate dementia. Both groups were already being treated with a medication to enhance the availability of acetylcholine. Six hundred milligrams of alpha-lipoic acid was added to the treatment. The conclusion was that the rate of progression in the mild-dementia group was significantly slowed. The alpha-lipoic acid seemed to have no impact on the group with moderate dementia. In my opinion, this makes sense. The more damaged the neurons, the more difficult it would be to repair or prevent deterioration.

Epigallocatechin-3-gallate

Epigallocatechin-3-gallate is an antioxidant that is found in high amounts in green and black tea. Of course, it is present in other plants as well. This antioxidant has been the buzz of the town for many things, from weight loss to decreasing the risk of certain cancers.

As you have come to expect from me, the question I strive to answer is how does it work? After all, nothing is a panacea, and if we have even a basic understanding of the mechanism of action, or how it works, then we can be in a positon to make more informed decisions. What I know for sure is that there are always individuals and companies waiting on the sidelines to turn even the most promising research into snake oil and fairy dust, promising everything from a cure for cancer to turning you into Benjamin Button. My hope is that taking even a little time to understand what it takes to keep your body healthy, and how nutrients and lifestyle can complement that, will put you in the driver's seat when it comes to your health and well-being.

So what have we learned about the power of tea so far? A study published in the *Journal of Nutrition, Health, and Aging* in 2016 followed a group of 957 seniors from 2003 to 2010. Every two years, they collected data on their lifestyles, medical conditions, exercise, and socialization habits. They also performed a standardized cognitive test on the subjects. After correcting for a series of variables, they came to the conclusion that just one cup of tea daily decreased the risk of declining cognitive function by 50 percent. They also noted that if the individual carried the gene that increased the risk of developing Alzheimer's disease (APOE e4 gene), then that risk was decreased by 86 percent.

To help elucidate the mechanism of action, researchers used animal models (mice) that were infected with a precursor to the human beta-amyloid protein that is found in high concentrations in the brain of individuals with Alzheimer's disease. This beta-amyloid protein is thought to contribute to the damage found in the brain of

Alzheimer's patients. Researchers found that EGCG played a role in promoting an enzyme that was able to help prevent the formation of this destruction protein. They postulated that EGCG could play a role in preventing the development of this dreaded form of dementia.

So how many cups of tea a day does it take to keep dementia away? A single cup of tea may contain from one hundred to two hundred milligrams of EGCG. It has not been determined the amount that would be the most effective. I would postulate that, like most things, the amount would depend on the individual. If you have the genetics of a "superager" (yes, that is a term), then you may be more resilient than if you carry the gene that increases the risk of dementia. I would say that one to two cups a day sounds like a reasonable approach given that the study mentioned above looked at individuals who consumed at least one cup a day.

Brain Exercises

We have discussed the impact of physical exercise on the brain, but can brain function be improved with mental gymnastics?

It makes intuitive sense that the more we use our brain to learn, process, and solve challenges, the more accessible it would seem to us. Do you remember going back to school after a long, lazy summer break, where your goal was to utilize as little brain power as possible? How did you feel that first week going back to school when you were expected to be all caught up on Algebra I so you could move on to Algebra II? A bit of a struggle, right? After all, how many of us spent any time reviewing math over the summer? Simply stated, you use it, or you lose it! Having said that, are there particular forms of brain exercises that seem to work better than others? Many researchers are working on this very question, and so far, a few things seem to be ahead of the pack.

Dual N-Back to Improve Memory

There are two main cognitive brain-training programs that researchers use to evaluate cognitive function, "dual n-back" and "complex span." Researchers at Johns Hopkins University found that the dual n-back training program was capable of improving functioning memory by a whopping 30 percent while increasing brain activity in the prefrontal cortex, the area of the brain that plays a significant role in learning.

So what is dual n-back? As the name implies, in this training exercise, the individual is exposed to two stimuli simultaneously, one visual and the other auditory. These sequences build on each other, and the individual then has to recall if the current sequence is the same one presented one, two, three, or even four rounds back. As you can imagine, this can be pretty challenging, but Johns Hopkins University was able to show that just one month of doing this daily enhances memory by up to 30 percent! Sign me up as soon as the consumer version becomes available.

Turning down the amygdala with neurofeedback

What if you can train the brain to treat itself? Imagine being able to treat stress and anxiety by simply feeding back the signal that part of the brain needs to self-soothe. Is this magic or the promising science of neurofeedback?

One of the challenges researchers have encountered in developing effective neurofeedback strategies is the ability to monitor the emotional center of the brain, the amygdala. If you could visualize

the activity of the amygdala during a high-anxiety moment, then

you would be able to provide an appropriate feedback stimulus that

would help to quiet the over-activity of that part of the brain,

thereby providing some relief to the individual.

According to the September 2016 issue of *Biological*

Psychiatry, it seems that researchers have developed a new, reliable

imaging tool that is able to provide neurofeedback from the

amygdala using EEG (electroencephalogram) monitoring. This is

how it would work—electrodes would be placed on the scalp that

would capture the electrical activity of the emotional center, the

amygdala. That electrical activity would then be converted into an

auditory stimulus or a noise—the louder the noise, the more chaotic

the electrical activity emanating from the amygdala. The individual

hooked up to the electrodes would then attempt to quiet the noise

using whatever technique (deep breathing, visualization, etc.) that

he or she found to be effective. The researchers found they were

able to train forty individuals to reduce the activity within the

amygdala. They also found the reduction of the activity in the amygdala corresponded with a change in emotional response to a stressful event.

Now imagine the potential of such a noninvasive tool to help us manage our stress. For example, I imagine a day that part of our school curriculum will be entitled "stress-resistance training." This course would include tools such as this one that would help us learn to mitigate the effect of stress on our health and well-being.

Meditation

I like to think of meditation as biofeedback without all the bells and whistles.

What's New on the Horizon?

There are so many ways that the brain is susceptible to damage, yet our tools for brain rescue seem to still be extremely limited. It seems that each day brings with it more and more individuals who are afflicted with neurodegenerative disorders. Are there new treatment modalities for protection or even reversal of damage looming on the horizon?

Stem Cells and Neurodegenerative Conditions

A neurodegenerative condition is a disorder where the neurons or cells in the nervous system degenerate or become damaged at an accelerated rate. The disorder that results depends on the area of the brain or spinal cord that is affected. Conditions that fall into this category are disorders such as Parkinson's, Alzheimer's, and even multiple sclerosis, which is also classified as an autoimmune condition. In all of these disorders, treatment options are limited, and there are currently no known cures. This can leave us feeling vulnerable and defenseless, as if waiting for the proverbial other shoe to drop squarely on our heads, turning us into helpless victims. This stress and panic increases even further if we witness our parents, or any close relative, struggle with any of these dreaded conditions. Even though these disorders affect millions of people and are projected to affect millions more as the population ages, we know there are numerous researchers and scientists tirelessly working to ensure that we can always live with dignity and grace.

Studies looking at mesenchymal stem cells are giving us hope in this direction. While it seems that we are just beginning to explore the potential of regenerative cellular therapy, the initial results are looking extremely promising. For example, there are several animal-model studies utilizing human mesenchymal stem cells that show that parts of the brain involved in depression, such as the hippocampus, can actually be regenerated, and that this regeneration correlates with an improvement in the depressive symptoms. Of course, these are not human studies, and the jury is still out, but to keep us optimistic about the future, I will list several of the studies that are currently stirring up a lot of questions.

In a study by Tfilin and others, published in *Molecular Psychiatry* in 2009, labeled adult mesenchymal stem cells were injected directly into the brain of the Flinders sensitive line, a rat animal model for depression. What they found were the rats that were injected with the mesenchymal stem cells showed significant improvement in behavioral performance. They found that this improvement in behavior correlated with the formation of new nerve cells in areas of the brain that were affected by depression, such as the hippocampus. They also found the labeled stem cells in these same areas of the brain.

Numerous other studies in animal models show that mesenchymal stem cells can activate cells in the brain that eat up substances in the brain that contribute to diseases, such as Alzheimer's and Parkinson's disease.

Well, injecting stem cells directly into the brain sounds a little harsh. Is there another delivery route that shows promise? Researchers at the University of Seoul in Korea radiolabeled human stem cells and injected them into a vein of the study animal every two weeks for anywhere from three to ten months. Their study found improvements in the ability to learn and the ability to remember. They also found important changes in the cytokine interleukin-10 that has an anti-inflammatory role in the body. Most importantly, the researchers were able to locate the labeled stem cells in the brain, suggesting that they can indeed cross the blood-brain barrier to enter into the brain to take effect.

Parting Words: My Personal "Keeping My Brain Happy" Routine

This is the part where I name names and invite you to take a look into my routine to give you an example of what putting together a routine may look like for yourself.

Now, fair warning, I do not presume to know where you are currently nor what is best for you physically or even mentally speaking. Only you and your physician can make that decision. That said, I hope my routine inspires you to find your own. I am going to share with you what makes me feel best.

This in no way implies that I do this 100 percent of the time. I am human, and some days get the best of me before I can get the best out of them. However, I feel my best when I am able to do these things consistently.

Now, for the routine: I wake up in the morning, hopefully after a good night's sleep, and I spend an extra five minutes in bed taking deep breaths. When I inhale, I make sure to appreciate all the good things in my life, and on exhalation, I express gratitude for the amazing day ahead of me.

Some days, it is more challenging than others, but this simple practice oftentimes puts my mind in a place to give more attention to the positive things that come my way and less attention to the things that seem to present themselves as obstacles.

Keep in mind, studies tell us that, as women, our brains are wired to give more attention to negative situations as opposed to our male counterparts, whose brains seem to be wired so positive events have more of an impact. This information just reiterates to me the importance of this morning routine.

Next, after my hygienic routine, I prepare myself a breakfast with lean proteins, vegetables, or fruits high in antioxidants and complex carbohydrates. My favorite breakfast is an egg white omelet with onions and peppers, along with one slice of whole-grain toast with fruit puree or a whey-concentrate protein shake.

After a routine like this, I am more than ready to face my day, feeling confident, powerful, and, yes, even sexy.

Sexercise:

A "Sexy Back" Activity

For this chapter's activity, use the blanks below to write down your morning routine. Now, be honest. No one's going to see this but you.

_____

_____

_____

_____

_____

_____

Okay, great. Now look for places to improve what you do every morning. For instance, if you notice a lot of fast, processed, microwave, or convenience food in your breakfast, find ways to replace those with "whole" foods, such as real eggs, fresh fruit, and vegetables.

Maybe it's your thoughts that are your undoing. When you wake up, what is the first thought that comes into your head? The thoughts you start the day with often set the tone for the rest of the day. This can be challenging, and one way to start changing this is by starting a gratitude journal. Before you get out of bed, write at least three things present in your life now that make you smile, that make you feel at peace, or that bring you a sense of gratitude.

Sometimes, we don't quite realize how bad our habits are until we stop, write them down, and look at them objectively.

Here is an example of a brain-boosting morning:

- Wake up with gradual lighting.
- Give thanks for three things in your life before getting out of bed.
- Take fifteen minutes to meditate.
- Take a twenty-minute walk.
- Eat a healthy breakfast—blueberry, nuts, oatmeal, or a cup of tea.

Chapter 3:

Sexy Hair—

Because You Are Worth It

"If you want to make a permanent change, stop focusing on the size of your problems and start focusing on the size of you!"

—T. Harv Eker

A woman's hair is often referred to as her "crowning glory." Now, this seemingly innocuous statement carries with it a host of societal and personal burdens that are often echoed around the world. As women, we oftentimes spend numerous hours talking, thinking, and strategizing about our hair.

If men think about sex approximately once an hour—according to an Ohio University study—women can sometimes easily double that amount of time thinking about their hair, especially if they are experiencing issues with hair loss, and a surprising number of women do over the age of forty. An article published in the journal *Social Science and Medicine* in 1994 noted that 88 percent of women experiencing issues with hair loss felt that it had a negative impact on their daily life. Seventy-five percent felt that it negatively impacted their self-esteem.

Why is our hair so important to us? It boils down to the simple matter of our hair being, well, not so simple. After all, this isn't just hair. Instead, we attach our sexuality, confidence, self-esteem, and even our femininity to our hair.

So whenever our hair starts experiencing any adverse reactions, such as falling out, breaking, frizzing, splitting at the ends, or turning gray, panic sets in because, to some of us, it is not just losing hair—it may begin to feel as if we are losing a crucial part of who we are as well.

The Hair: More than Meets the Eye

Let me start this chapter by saying, first and foremost, that our hair does *not* define who we are. We are, as I think we all suspect, much more than our appearance indicates and surely much more than a few thousand hair follicles dictate.

Therefore, hair loss—or even damage—does not make us less than who we really are and certainly not less than who we were meant to be. On many occasions, it may, however, define how we *think* about ourselves. As we've already discovered in this book so far, the way the world sees us oftentimes reflects the way we see ourselves.

So what to do? In this chapter, I will tell you not only what science says about your hair, but I will also share with you my personal struggles and the secrets I have discovered while writing the story of my hair. My goal is that by the end of this chapter, you will feel empowered to embark on your own personal, optimal hair program, whatever that may be.

Reaching Peace with Your Hair:

Step One: Put It in Perspective

I, too, have had to go through the emotional and physical ups and downs that accompany sudden and unexplained hair loss. So while I know that it is difficult, I am asking you to find a way to let go of some of the angst associated with whatever hair issues you are experiencing, and work on finding a place of acceptance. From this space, it is easier to get to a place where you can see the issues in a clearer, more focused, and more objective way. This then allows you to make the decision that puts your well-being as a top priority and start creating a plan that fits you.

So whether you choose to move forward by bonding with other women who may be experiencing similar issues, experimenting with wigs to spice up your looks, or setting aside some time each day to scream about it until you're hoarse, I urge you to find a way to come to a place of acceptance. Acceptance is not resignation or defeat, but rather, it is simply acknowledging what "is" now so you can focus on and identify what comes next. Acceptance empowers, while panic takes away that power, leaving you less focused on seeing the best path in front of you. Those with a lack of focus tend to "run around in circles." Most importantly, medically speaking, panic induces a sea of stress hormones that can only make the situation worse.

Step Two: Seek Help

Next, follow acceptance with action. If you are experiencing serious issues with your hair, visit your doctor as there are many medical conditions that can cause excessive hair loss. Conditions that can cause hair loss or thinning include, but are not limited to, the following:

- Hypothyroidism
- Adverse reactions to certain medications used to treat depression, heart issues, etc.
- Hyperparathyroidism
- Scalp infections, such as the fungal infection commonly referred to as ringworm
- Autoimmune conditions, such as alopecia areata and scleroderma
- Psoriasis
- Seborrheic dermatitis
- Stress
- Hairstyles that create excessive traction or pulling on the scalp

Step Three: Lifestyle and Hairstyle

Finally, learn about your hair. The more you know, the better a participant you are in your hair's recovery. Start by taking stock of all your hair products and habits. How many times do you do any chemical processing to your hair (color, perms, relaxers, and so on)? Are you using the right product for your hair type? Is your hairstyle potentially contributing to your hair issues? For example, hair loss can occur if hair is braided, pinned, or pulled back too tightly. This is referred to as traction alopecia. This kind of alopecia can then permanently scar the scalp, leaving it unable to regrow hair in the future. Discuss with your haircare specialist or dermatologist if any of these factors could be exacerbating your hair issues.

Take a close look at other lifestyle patterns, such as exercise, types of foods, and potentially toxic habits like smoking. Smoking constricts blood vessels, and this could potentially compromise blood flow to the hair, thus reducing delivery of those vital nutrients that the hair requires to thrive. Other ways smoking can lead to hair loss are by causing inflammation in the hair follicles and artificially lowering estrogen levels and increasing male hormones,

99

testosterone and dihyrotestosterone, associated with hair loss. Smokers may also be two and a half times more likely to have premature graying of the hair. Heavy drinking has also been associated with accelerated hair loss.

Finally, your emotional state or level of stress could be playing a role here, as well. A twin study done at Case Western Reserve University showed that this may be especially true for women. The study evaluated twins and their lifestyles while trying to adjust for other variables. What researchers noted was that twins in stable marriages had a fuller head of hair when compared to those in dysfunctional relationships or to those who had suffered the loss of a spouse. This may be yet another way that stress can negatively impact the quality of your life.

The Story of Your Hair: You're the Author, Not the Reader

Moving forward, I want you to think of your hair as a garden that produces an array of vibrant fruits and vegetables all in their season. Gardens require attention, care, nutrient-rich soil, and the appropriate amount of water in order to flourish and grow. These things must be administered at the right time and in the right amounts depending on the plant you are attempting to cultivate. For example, you would not place water onto the leaves of the plant in an attempt to provide water. You would ensure that the roots are firmly planted in soil that has just the right amount of moisture. So it is with your hair. You have to feed the hair from the inside out.

What Is in a Hair? The Three Distinct Layers of Hair

The hair consists primarily of a protein called keratin. This is the same protein that is found abundantly in nails and the outer layer of the skin. Three percent of the hair shaft is made up of fatty acids. Each strand of hair has three distinct layers:

- **The medulla:** The innermost layer of the hair follicle is called the medulla, which is present in thick hairs.

- **The cortex:** The middle layer is called the cortex. It is this layer that provides our hair with its texture and color. This is the layer that also determines how strong the hair is.

- **The cuticle:** Finally, the protective layer most of us are familiar with is called the cuticle.

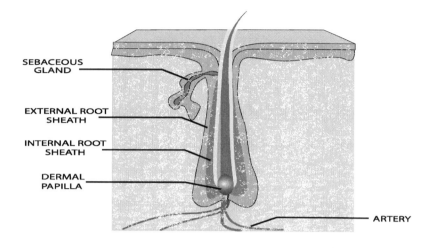

SEBACEOUS GLAND

EXTERNAL ROOT SHEATH

INTERNAL ROOT SHEATH

DERMAL PAPILLA

ARTERY

Figure 3.1: *Structure of the hair root; it's more than meets the eye.*

As you can see from Figure 3.1, the hair root is below the surface of the skin and is surrounded by the follicle. At the bottom of the hair follicle is a structure called the dermal papilla. The blood vessels supplying nutrients to the hair follicle come in through this structure. The dermal papilla is also the center of hormonal interaction with the hair. For example, excessive male hormones can act on this part of the follicle to cause thinning of the hair follicle and the hair, eventually leading to hair loss and even balding.

How Does Your Garden Grow? The Three Cycles of Hair Growth

Now that we know what makes up our hair, let's see how our garden grows. The hair has three cycles of growth:

1. **Anagen phase:** This is referred to as the active growth phase. About 90 percent of the hair is in this phase at all times. This phase lasts between two and seven years.

2. **Catagen phase:** This is often referred to as the transition stage because hair is transitioning from the active to the resting phase. This stage tells us that active hair growth is coming to an end. This phase lasts approximately two to three weeks. It is in this phase when the blood supply is cut off from the follicle, and the hair enters the next stage.

3. **Telogen or resting phase:** During this phase, the hair does not grow because it is detached from its blood supply, and the hair sheds. Roughly 10 percent of hair is in this stage at any given time. This stage can last up to five to six weeks. After this stage, the follicle rejoins its blood supply, and a new hair begins to grow, thus starting the cycle over again.

Hair can grow approximately ten centimeters per year (roughly four inches). This is an average, and some people's hair can grow even faster than this. We lose an average of one hundred hairs per day. On days that we wash our hair, that increases to about 250 hairs during the "lather, rinse, and repeat" process. To give some perspective, we have about 120,000 to 150,000 strands of hair imbedded in our scalp. As you can see, if the cycle proceeds as planned, we should have plenty of hair to last us a lifetime.

The figure below shows how we lose our hair:

Hair Loss

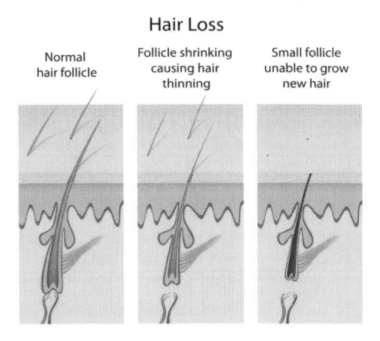

Figure 3.2: *Follicle pulling away from dermal papilla.*

How to Grow Your Garden: Hair Care for the Careful Gardener

Now that we understand a bit about how our hair grows, it's time to explore ways to best nourish and grow our hair. Factors such as nutrient deficiencies, environmental pollution, lifestyle habits, medications, styling and processing of hair, excessive exposure to heat, excessive exposure to UV radiation from the sun, hormonal changes, aging, genetics, and medical conditions can negatively impact the health of the hair. Let's approach it in several stages and address each stage in more detail.

The First Stage: Evaluation

First, evaluate your diet and lifestyle habits. Take a good look at how you eat, sleep, work, and live, and then ask yourself the following questions:

- **Is your diet supplying the nutrients you need to support healthy hair growth?** Remember, healthy hair starts from within.

- **Have you done a lot of crash or yo-yo dieting?** If so, keep in mind the effects may not be seen for up to three to six months.

- **Are you vegan or vegetarian?** All of these factors can cause a relative protein or nutrient deficiency that can cause hair loss.

- **Are you constantly under severe stress, or have you recently experienced a traumatic event or illness?** In this case, hair loss may continue for eight to twelve months.

- **Do you smoke or consume excessive alcohol?** This can lead to excessive hair loss and premature graying of the hair.

  Knowing that your diet, lifestyle, or stress level may be damaging your hair is a great way to begin to isolate the problem.

The Second Stage: Hair-Care Routine

Next, explore your hair-care routine. Look at what you do on a daily basis, and try to determine if this routine is helping or hurting the growth of your hair. These are some questions you may ask yourself:

- How often do you perform some processing on your hair?

- Do you perm, relax, or color?

- Do you often wear your hair in tight ponytails, braids, or curlers?

- What types of shampoos do you use?

- How often do you shampoo?

- Do you condition your hair?

Over treating your hair, using harsh shampoos or conditioners, and perpetually twisting or tightening your hair can do damage that can lead to permanent hair loss or simply unhealthy hair. Less can be more. See if you can limit the amount of processing. Yes, we may be not ready to let our gray hairs show, but coloring too frequently may leave us without any hair to color. Try using powders or sticks that temporarily camouflage grays so that you don't have to color as frequently. Speak with your hair-care specialist about coloring products that may be gentler on the hair. Avoid combining processing procedures, such as relaxing and coloring, at the same appointment. Limit styling your hair with high-heat appliances. Occasionally let your hair air dry. Speak with your stylist about products that make this process possible.

The Third Stage: Look at Your Medicine Cabinet

Next, take stock of your medication and supplement list. For example, did you know that too much vitamin A or the mineral selenium can actually cause hair thinning and loss? Certain medications or drugs can cause the hair to go into the resting phase too early, thus causing excessive shedding. This can occur weeks or even months after starting the medication. Some examples of drugs that can contribute to excessive hair loss are thyroid medications, acne medications with vitamin A, cholesterol-lowering drugs, antiseizure medications, and blood pressure medications to name a few. Speak with your doctor or pharmacist about your medication and supplements and their potential side effects.

The Fourth Stage: Medical Evaluation

Finally, try to rule out medical causes for any potential hair loss. You can start by visiting your doctor for an assessment. While menopause and the hormonal changes that accompany it may increase a woman's risk of experiencing accelerated hair loss, menstruating women can also be at an increased risk due to excessive blood loss, leading to iron deficiency and anemia. Remember, iron in red blood cells helps to supply nutrients and oxygen to the hair follicle. Without a steady supply of nutrients, the hair follicle will prematurely die, leading to increased shedding.

Menopause and Hair Loss

Many women over the age of forty experience some hair thinning, hair loss, and hair-texture changes. As women transition through menopause, many of these changes start becoming more noticeable. In fact, menopause can leave many women pondering why, as they get older, hair seems to migrate from the scalp into the chin. Even though women who are experiencing these changes do not need studies to confirm the obvious, researchers have indeed found that this pattern of hair developing a fondness for the chin as we age is a very real phenomenon in many women. It was observed that the endocrine changes associated with menopausal aging can cause up to a twentyfold increase in chin hair and a twofold increase in hair on the upper lip.

These external manifestations may trigger issues that can bring us to a crossroad in our lives. After all, living and aging in a culture that constantly bombards us with images and messages of what it should look and feel like to be sexy, vibrant, and confident, very few of us will escape unscathed. The message that we are not enough unless we fit into a certain image has already permeated the very fiber of our being. How do we resolve these conflicting images of who we should be and whom we have become? After all, this is the time in our lives when we have gathered enough experience, wisdom, and self-knowledge to feel confident expressing who we are, what we want, and how we want our life to develop. Now, when we look in the mirror and notice the thinning hair on our scalp and the excess hair on our face, we are forced to confront that lingering message from our youth that getting older makes us somehow "less than."

I challenge you to reject this message by understanding that the changes that occur as we get older are part of a biological process and not a statement on your right to be fully you. Understanding the process puts us in charge of making the choices that support us in being the healthiest and sexiest version of ourselves.

The Process

Excess testosterone is thought to play a role in contributing to this pattern of hair baldness and seeming redistribution. But before we go vilifying testosterone and making this a simple "open-and-shut case", researchers have discovered that certain women with low testosterone and normal BMI (body mass index) actually regrew scalp hair with testosterone-replacement therapy. This study, published in the *British Journal of Dermatology* in February 2012, demonstrated hair regrowth in 63 percent of the women involved. It was noted that the women who did not regrow hair had much higher BMIs than the women who did. The researchers speculated that one possible cause of this noted effect may be attributable to testosterone's anabolic property, or the ability to make things such as muscles or even hair grow.

Of course, more research will be needed before this question can be answered definitively. One thing I know for sure is that many women would gladly take the wisdom that comes with age but willingly pass on the excess facial hair that seems to want to tag along for the ride. I believe that as the story of hair loss unravels, we will find many contributors to this saga—from nutritional deficiencies to hormonal culprits, environmental toxins, and psychological and physical stressors.

Other Causes of Hair Loss

We are now beginning to scratch the surface as to why some people seem destined to lose hair, while others seem to be able to hold on to a full head of hair well into their golden years. We understand that there are some genetic contributors, but what are the changes that seem to be directly responsible for hair loss and thinning? We have heard of male pattern baldness and female pattern baldness, but what do these really mean? Are the mechanisms behind male and female pattern baldness similar or as different as night and day? Most importantly, is there anything that can be done to stabilize or even reverse this process?

Androgenic Alopecia: Male Pattern Baldness

Although this is commonly referred to as male pattern baldness, it can affect both men and women. It is thought to be a genetically programmed pattern of hair loss. Individuals with this pattern of hair loss can start seeing these changes as early as their early twenties or even late teens. This pattern of hair loss is characterized by gradual receding of the hairline with the most noticeable hair loss at the crown and frontal areas. Women tend to experience this later on in life, such as in their forties, and there tends to be a more generalized thinning that accompanies this pattern.

There are several factors that are thought to contribute to this pattern of hair loss. Many of us are familiar with the theory that hormones play a role. It is thought that a potent form of the male hormone testosterone called dihydrotestosterone (DHT) causes the hair follicle to prematurely enter into the resting phase, thus leading to hair loss. Some research suggests that this happens because DHT causes the increase of a substance called transforming growth factor beta-2, known to be toxic to the hair follicle in vitro.

Researchers may have stumbled upon another contributor to this problem that can plague men and women alike. They found that the scalps of bald men have an excessive amount of prostaglandin D2, a protein that blocks the growth of the hair follicle. So, already, you can see that there are at least two substances that have the potential to contribute to accelerated hair loss. Also note that each substance seems to have a different mechanism of action. DHT seems to put the follicle into the catagen phase, while prostaglandin D2 acts by directly blocking the growth of the follicle. This, once again, seems to support one of my core beliefs—very seldom is there an isolated cause, and therefore, very seldom will there be an isolated solution.

Involutional Alopecia

Simply put, this is the thinning of the hair that often accompanies aging. In this condition, more of the hair follicles can abruptly transition from the growth phase into the resting phase, leading to increased hair loss. Hairs can also become significantly shorter as they are now spending a much shorter time in the growth phase.

Alopecia Areata / Alopecia Universalis

In this section, it may seem to some as if I have gone into too many details, and it may even seem overwhelming at some points. If, however, you have experienced the destruction of self-confidence and hopelessness this condition can trigger, you may begin to understand my desire to offer real scientific hope and a basic understanding of the pathology of this form of alopecia. I believe that knowledge and understanding oftentimes lead to empowerment and hope, thus giving us the foundation we need for confidence.

So what is alopecia? Alopecia areata is the type of hair loss that often starts suddenly and leaves sufferers with patchy hair loss throughout the scalp. Oftentimes, the trigger is not identified. If the hair loss results in total baldness, then it is referred to as alopecia totalis. If the condition affects all the hair on the body, including the eyebrows, axillary, and pubic hair, then it is referred to as alopecia universalis. While it occurs commonly in young adults and children, it can also affect adults at any age. The good news here is that about 90 percent of the people suffering from mild to moderate alopecia areata will regrow some or all of their hair.

Alopecia areata is a disorder of the hair follicle cycling phases. In this condition, the body's immune cells are somehow triggered to attack the bulb of hairs that are in the anagen, or growth, phase, thus triggering the abrupt loss of anagen hairs. This attack by the body's own immune system classifies this disorder as an autoimmune condition. This theory is supported by the fact that in quite a few instances, this form of alopecia is often associated with other autoimmune conditions, such as eczema, Hashimoto's thyroiditis, vitiligo, and pernicious anemia. Recent work on this disorder is beginning to identify some of the immune cells involved in this condition. This offers hope to the 10 percent of those individuals who do not experience spontaneous regrowth of the hair or who are suffering from a severe form of this disease.

The immune system is indeed a complicated system. When it is working optimally, we are blissfully unaware of the symphony that it takes to keep us healthy and balanced. However, if we were to take a closer look at all the different types of immune cells that it takes to run the show, we would immediately become overwhelmed and wonder how in the world this many cells can work together in harmony to keep us well. Even seasoned immunologists who work daily on deciphering the immune system do not have all the answers. So my goal here is not to throw complicated information your way but, rather, to try to present a simplified, basic version of how the immune system works and some ways that it can malfunction and contribute to diseases such as the autoimmune disorder alopecia areata.

The primary goal of the immune system is to be ready to fight, sequester, or divert anything in the body that cannot be identified as "self." If it is not "self," it must be sequestered or removed as it is considered a potential threat. In the case of viruses, bacteria, and even cancer cells—"self" that has become dysregulated—this can be a life-saving intervention. However, if the immune system starts to identify "self" as the enemy, this can create a myriad of issues depending on the organ system or tissue that is impacted.

It was noted by some researchers that T lymphocytes, an important part of the immune system, play a role in alopecia areata. These T lymphocytes are often commonly called T helper cells. The role of T helper cells is to recognize foreign antigens and to secrete inflammatory substances called cytokines that then trigger other T cells and B cells to mount a response against the invaders. Generally speaking, there are two basic categories of T helper cells: T helper cells that activate other T cells to help destroy infected cells, and T helper cells that amplify B cells to form antibodies to fight infection in the blood or other bodily fluids.

T helper cells are activated when they bind to an antigen-presenting cell (APC). This simply means that there are specialized cells in the immune system that capture the foreign substance or antigen and present it to the T helper cells, so they can bind to the antigen and start getting the body ready to fight off the invader. The antigen-presenting cells bind the antigen using a protein on the surface called the MHC (major histocompatibility complex). If all is working well, then the antigen presented is indeed an invader, and steps are taken to eliminate it. If, however, the antigen presented is an autoantigen or "self," such as the hair follicle, then accelerated hair loss occurs.

In alopecia areata, researchers found a significantly increased number of T helper cells at the base of the hair follicle. This indicates that the immune cells have determined that the hair follicle is a foreign substance or an invader and have set out on a mission to destroy it. The epithelium of the growing hair follicle usually enjoys immune-privileged status because the inner root and shaft do not express the MHC protein that allows the antigen to bind. This means that the hair follicle is not normally targeted by the immune system. In alopecia areata, there seems to be a mechanism that increases the expression of MHC in the hair follicle, thus making it a target for the T cells.

T helper cells use different messengers called cytokines to stimulate the other cells to produce even more inflammatory substances. One such pathway involves the activation of a specific enzyme called the Janus kinase (JAK) enzyme. This enzyme then triggers several reactions that cause the cells to produce even more products of inflammation. Small trials treating alopecia universalis with immune-suppression drugs that inhibit the JAK enzyme (JAK inhibitors) have had promising results with regrowth of hair, thus, once again, supporting the role of inflammatory cytokines in this process. These drugs are already in use for treating other autoimmune conditions such as rheumatoid arthritis.

As if this weren't complicated enough, other potential contributors are being explored. Research points to more potential aggravators such as intense emotional stress, infectious entities like cytomegalovirus and scalp fungi, and even genetic susceptibility. Certain genetic markers seem to be linked to the susceptibility and severity of the disorder. However, like most genetic situations, environmental triggers play an important role. I would posit that the above mentioned potential aggravators can act as potential triggers in susceptible individuals. In my opinion, expecting autoimmune disorders to only have one trigger is something that we seem to struggle with in the scientific community. Therefore, we are often tempted to completely disregard research that appears to be contradictory instead of exploring the possibility that both results may exist in certain circumstances.

For example, some studies show a significant link between intense emotional stress and alopecia areata, while others do not support this link. This is not necessarily contradictory. Perhaps some people are more genetically susceptible to this environmental trigger. An article published in the *American Journal of Pathology* in December 2007 offers up a mechanism on how neurochemical changes that can occur during extremely stressful situations, can impact the hair follicle. Human hair follicles were exposed to substance P, a neuropeptide produced in high amounts during a high-stress response. They found that the affected hair follicles were pushed into an early catagen phase. They also noted an upregulation in the MHC class I immunoreactivity, an indication that the hair follicles were losing their immune-privileged status, thus making them susceptible to an autoimmune response.

If we understand and accept that there seem to be multiple mechanisms involved in this form or any form of hair loss, then it allows us to be patient with ourselves when we begin the journey to maximize our hair's potential. We now understand that sometimes it may require trials of different treatment options as we work on discovering the mechanism behind our hair loss. We also begin to realize that with all imbalances, we need to examine all areas of our lives.

Scarring Alopecia

This condition is due to inflammatory skin conditions that cause scarring of the scalp, leading to permanent hair loss. Skin infections and conditions such as lupus, lichen planus, and acne keloidalis can lead to scarring alopecia. The underlying pattern of scarring alopecia is the oftentimes irreversible destruction of the hair follicles, leaving in their place scar tissue. Sometimes, the affected areas can appear smooth and patchy, similar to alopecia areata. In scarring alopecia, however, the edges of the patch oftentimes appear more irregular. At times, depending on what condition is triggering this type of alopecia, the scalp may appear red, scaly, or even pustular. Oftentimes, to get a definitive diagnosis, a scalp biopsy is performed. Frequently, inflammation is found at the base of the hair follicles.

If scarring alopecia is caught prior to the permanent destruction of the hair follicles, then your dermatologist may inject steroids into the lesions in an attempt to reduce and calm the inflammatory process, thus giving the hair follicles an opportunity to recover. Other potential treatment modalities include antibiotics and isotretinoin, a form of vitamin A. If you suspect you may have this condition, a visit to your dermatologist is in order.

What about Gray Hair?

We have all been witness to people who seem to gray prematurely. In fact, one of my high school classmates had about 30 percent gray hair, and I remembered thinking, "Maybe he is older than he looks, or he is under a lot of stress." Those two thoughts probably sum up what gray hair signifies to many people: aging or stressing. But what really causes hair to turn gray?

If you recall, I alluded to one possible cause earlier when I mentioned that individuals with higher levels of oxidative stress seem to be at increased risk for premature graying of the hair. There is one theory that seems to be consistent with the mechanism of why hair turns gray. This mechanism suggests that hair is being bleached from inside the body. The body produces hydrogen peroxide as a byproduct or waste product of many of its reactions. This production of hydrogen peroxide occurs in the hair roots, as well. When we are younger, we have an abundance of an enzyme called catalase, whose job it is to break down the excess hydrogen peroxide into harmless water and oxygen. As we get older—and perhaps more stressed—our body makes less of this enzyme, and hydrogen peroxide builds up in the hair follicles, bleaching the hair from the inside out. This seems to be at least part of the story of gray hair.

There are some reversible causes of gray hair, including vitamin B_{12} deficiency or problems with the thyroid gland. When treated, the pigment gradually returns to the hair. For many of us, however, genetics also play a large role in when and how much gray hair we exhibit.

Where Is the Cure?

Now that we know the cause, is there a cure? That answer may be a resounding yes, according to some published studies. Research looking at a product called PC-KUS, or pseudocatalase, looks promising. It seems that applying this product topically to the hair and scalp may actually help return some of the natural color to the hair by destroying hydrogen peroxide in the hair follicles. This product seems to require activation by a special light in order to work. Before you go rushing out to purchase this product, be aware that you can fall into the trap of buying from disreputable sources as this product does not seem to be readily available yet.

There are other possibilities on the horizon. Researchers at New York University Medical Center have located a special protein that seems to help coordinate the stem cells that give hair its color (melanocytes). This special protein is called WNT protein, and as usual, the story is much more complicated than simply "apply here." Bottom line, we are perhaps the closest we have ever been to the Holy Grail of preventing or reversing gray hair. But, would we want to?

What Now?

Now that you have taken stock of your lifestyle habits and hair care and obtained a medical evaluation, what's next? Next is putting together a plan that targets your areas of concern. If you have a medical condition, such as hypothyroidism or hyperparathyroidism, that can be treated, treat it. Keep in mind that part of treating any condition is creating the supporting lifestyle and dietary changes. After all, a healthy diet is the most important ingredient for maintaining a healthy head of hair.

Let's say that you lost your hair secondary to a thyroid condition that you have now corrected. Now, you are ready to regrow a new set of tresses. Now, it is time to remember what hair needs to grow and to be healthy and, subsequently, create the conditions that would support healthier hair growth. If we recall, the hair is made up of about 97 percent protein and 3 percent fatty acids. If we also recall, 90 percent of the hair is in the growing phase at any given time. Wow, a lot of fertilizer required indeed! Think about it, if there are not enough nutrients, including protein or good fats, then it would seem logical that more hair would go into the resting phase, thus leading to more hair loss and shedding.

Below, I will discuss certain nutrients that have been shown to have an impact on hair health. I will also address current treatments for particular conditions and will also touch on what is on the horizon—perhaps closer than we think—to help, maybe even regrow, a healthy head of hair. How exciting it is to live in the age of discovery!

Nutrients and the Hair

What are the nutrients that have been shown to contribute to healthy hair? The final jury is still out on the story of our hair, but thanks to diligent researchers, I am able to provide you with some tantalizing tidbits about keeping your hair well-nourished and healthy. As mentioned previously, hair is made up primarily of protein and is nourished via blood vessels carrying nutrients and hormones to the follicles. So let's explore some of the nutrients that seem to play an important role in maintaining healthy hair. Keep in mind, the foundation is always a healthy diet.

Iron and Healthy Hair

Over forty years of research has linked iron deficiency with hair loss. Recent studies suggest that iron deficiency can contribute to hair loss even in the absence of anemia. Lack of iron seems to put more hair into the telogen, or resting phase.

Now, before you run out and start supplementing with iron, get your levels checked by your physician. The story of iron is a little more complicated than "take iron to make hair grow." If there is an iron deficiency, you and your doctor can work to determine the cause. In menstruating women, the most common cause is heavy or excessive bleeding during menstruation. Be aware that there are other causes of iron deficiency, such as iron-deficient diets (like an imbalanced, vegetarian diet), decreased absorption, as can be seen in excessive use of antacids and H_2 blockers, and medical conditions like celiac disease and occult bleeding, as possible in colon cancer. Some signs of iron deficiency, other than hair loss, can be fatigue, mental fogginess, an inflamed tongue, craving crunchy things (pica), anemia, and difficulty maintaining body temperature.

Another thing to be aware of is that excess iron is inflammatory to the body and can cause serious side effects. This is another reason to avoid blindly supplementing with iron before knowing your iron levels. Studies that investigated how little iron is too little suggest that individuals with ferritin levels less than forty may be more susceptible. Your doctor may want to perform a more comprehensive iron panel as ferritin levels can be impacted by things other than iron stores. For example, increased inflammation in the body can artificially elevate ferritin levels, giving the impression of normal iron storage when you may, indeed, have an iron deficiency. I would also like to reiterate here that while an iron deficiency may lead to anemia, anemia is not a required laboratory finding to diagnose iron deficiency. So have that discussion with your physician.

Vitamin C and Hair Loss—the Story of Antioxidants

Oxidative stress and free radicals have long been associated with accelerating the ageing process, and hair loss and graying are no exception. Free radicals are unstable molecules that can directly damage cells and our DNA. As we age, the rate of free radical production increases, and our body's ability to squelch their damage decreases. When this happens to the hair and scalp, it can result in the acceleration of thinning and graying of the hair. For example, dermal papillae from the balding scalp have been shown to contain higher levels of markers for DNA and oxidative stress damage when compared with dermal papillae from the non- balding scalp. The body naturally defends itself from free radicals with antioxidants, such as vitamins C and E, glutathione, and enzymes like superoxide dismutase, catalase, and glutathione peroxidase that break down waste products that can damage the body. So a deficiency in any of these natural antioxidants could, potentially, lead to issues with maintaining a healthy head of hair.

Topical Applications

How promising are topical applications? The jury is still out on this subject. However, several small studies give us some hope for the future as researchers continue to unravel the story of our hair.

Where possible, I will discuss the possible mechanism of action of these compounds. Understanding is the key to incorporating.

- **Melatonin:** Melatonin is the hormone in the body that helps us fall asleep more easily and helps regulate our sleep, wake cycle, or circadian rhythm. But what does melatonin have to do with hair? Interestingly, several studies show that the application of melatonin to the scalp may actually help reduce hair loss in androgenic alopecia. Why would this be? As mentioned previously, oxidative damage has been suggested as one of the major causes of premature hair loss and thinning. Melatonin, through its potent antioxidant ability, may just prevent some of this damage from occurring.

- **Topical procyanidin B-2, extracted from apples:** This antioxidant, extracted from apples, has been shown in studies to increase hair thickness and influence regrowth.

- **Adenosine:** Another topical application shown to have some effect is topical adenosine. A study done in Japan showed that this substance was able to increase the thickness of hair.

The challenge with all of these products is that they do not seem to be readily available to the consumer in a reliable form.

- **Ketoconazole:** A more easily accessible product that has shown some efficacy in reducing hair loss is ketoconazole, an antifungal found in many antidandruff shampoos, such as Nizoral. While the mechanism of action is unknown, one theory is that it may reduce inflammation in the scalp, thus decreasing repetitive insult to the hair follicles. Also, remember in previous alopecia areata discussions that it was theorized that infectious etiology could contribute to some cases of alopecia areata.

- **Caffeine:** Can you wake your hair up with a "cup of joe?" Well, science is suggesting this might just be the case. But before you go out on a coffee binge, just know that to get this effect you would have to drink about five hundred cups of coffee daily to achieve any hair benefits. Fortunately for us, the study shows that the topical application of coffee may actually stimulate hair growth. In this study, both male and female hair follicles were placed in a medium that contained caffeine. Caffeine was able to keep the hair in the growth phase (anagen) for a longer period of time, while accelerating the growth of the hair.

How is caffeine able to accomplish this feat? It seems that caffeine's effect on a certain protein called transforming growth factor beta-2 (TGF-beta2) may play a role. TGF-beta2, when present in high amounts in the dermal papillae that supply nutrients to the hair follicles, has the ability to put the hair follicle prematurely into the resting, or catagen, phase, thus leading to excessive hair loss. Caffeine seems to possess the capacity to suppress the formation of TGF-beta2.

Interestingly, this same study also showed that testosterone accelerated the formation of TGF-beta2 in male hair follicles but not in female hair follicles. This could help explain, based on the aforementioned study, why some women may actually regrow hair with testosterone instead of losing hair.

However, if we recall from the study, women with elevated BMIs, or who were significantly overweight, did not experience hair regrowth. Why would that be? One possible explanation could be tied to the fact that other researchers discovered that it is testosterone's conversion to the powerful dihydrotestosterone (DHT) that leads to the increased formation of TGF-beta2 in the root of the hair follicle and, ultimately, to the follicle's demise. The enzyme in the body that is responsible for this conversion is called 5-alpha reductase. Research tells us that high insulin levels found in conditions such as polycystic ovarian syndrome and insulin resistance can increase the levels of 5-alpha reductase, thus potentially leading to the formation of higher levels of DHT in the tissues. Many overweight individuals tend to also have accompanying insulin-management and glucose-intolerance issues, thus, potentially, leading to higher insulin levels and higher DHT levels, causing hair to be put into an early resting phase. Even though this is a theory, it is not too difficult to see the possibility of such an occurrence.

Medical Interventions

- **Topical minoxidil:** Minoxidil is a medication that was initially used in the 1970s to treat high blood pressure. It was noted that some individuals treated with this medication developed excessive hair growth as a common side effect. Hair regrowth was even noticed in male pattern baldness. Investigators then wondered if you could put this medication directly on the area that you wanted to treat. This would reduce the potential side effects of taking the medication systemically, while providing hair growth in the targeted areas; thus, topical minoxidil was born.

  How this drug works is still poorly understood, but it seems to be able to prolong the anagen (growth) phase while shortening the telogen (hair loss) phase and increase the diameter of the hair shaft. The most common side effects of topical minoxidil may be itching, dryness, and burning of the scalp. Of course, there is always the possibility that you may have an allergic reaction, as with any medication. Minoxidil seems to be more effective in androgenic alopecia than alopecia areata but is, at times, used for both.

- **Corticosteroids:** Corticosteroids are often used as a first-line treatment in alopecia areata. Steroids help decrease inflammation and reduce the immune response. Steroids can be applied topically or injected directly into the affected area of the scalp. In specially selected cases, steroids may be used systemically, but because of the much higher risk of systemic side effects, this option is usually not the first choice. Also, it was noted that there was a high rate of relapse when a systemic corticosteroid was discontinued.

- **Propecia:** Propecia is a medication specifically developed to treat a balding scalp or androgenic alopecia. It was discovered that the follicles of a balding scalp had a higher concentration of a hormone called DHT, or dihydrotestosterone. This hormone is produced when the sex hormone testosterone is acted upon by a specific enzyme called type II 5-alpha reductase. DHT is thought to cause shrinkage of the hair follicle, thus cutting off blood supply to the hair and, ultimately, leading to hair loss.

Propecia prevents testosterone from being converted into DHT, thus decreasing the concentration of DHT in the scalp. Propecia is used primarily in the male population. A few studies on postmenopausal females have shown it not to be effective for hair regrowth in women, or that the dosage in women needs to be higher for it to have any effect.

A few studies suggest that the blood pressure medicine spironolactone may have some efficacy in the female population, even if they do not have elevated male (androgenic) hormone levels. Clearly, you would need to have a conversation with your doctor to determine if any of these treatments would be appropriate for you.

- **Immunosuppressant Drugs:** Different forms of immunosuppressant medications have been noted to promote hair growth as an incidental side effect. The issue is a compromised immune system and the side effects that can

137

accompany significant suppression of the immune system. Two particular drugs, ruxolitinib and tofacitinib, that are approved by the FDA to control the immune system in other conditions, are currently being tested in patients with moderate to severe alopecia areata. These drugs belong to a class of medications referred to as JAK inhibitors. If we recall, the JAK enzymes are involved in a cascade that upregulates the immune system and increases inflammatory cytokines.

A small clinical study, sponsored by Columbia University in New York, had success not only in regrowth of hair but also in retention of hair once the treatment was terminated. We look forward to a larger study that can provide more insight and delineate safety measures. Interestingly, Mother Nature may be offering her version of a JAK inhibitor, at least according to some researchers. There are several studies looking at the curcumin mechanism of action that point to it being an inhibitor of the JAK-STAT pathway that seems to be a contributor to alopecia areata. Does this mean that curcumin potentially could be used as an adjunct in this disheartening condition? I am not aware of any large-scale studies looking at this question, but flavoring your food with a little extra turmeric may go well beyond flavor.

Stem Cells and Hair Regrowth

Recently, treatment with mesenchymal stem cells is being mentioned as one weapon in the arsenal against hair loss. But is there any evidence to support this being an effective treatment? Several studies seem to lend credence to the possibility that this may be an additional tool to consider. In September 2013, researchers Trink, Sorbellini, and others published a randomized, double-blind placebo study in the *British Journal of Dermatology* evaluating the effects of platelet-rich plasma (a source of mesenchymal stem cells) on alopecia areata. Forty-five patients with alopecia areata were enrolled in the study. They were randomly assigned to receive platelet-rich plasma (PRP), triamcinolone, or a placebo injected into a lesion on one half of the scalp. The other half of the scalp was left untreated. They received three treatments separated by one month. The researchers found that PRP increased hair regrowth to a significant extent, and this was followed by a reduction of itching and burning of the scalp. The pros of this potential treatment are that PRP is obtained from the patient, so there is no chance of rejection. Also, the potential downside of immunosuppressive therapy is avoided.

Another study exploring the potential mechanism of the action of PRP was published in the *Journal of Dermatologic Surgery* in July 2002. Using in vitro (in the laboratory) and in vivo (live animal studies), researchers were able to identify that there was a faster conversion from the telogen phase to the anagen phase. Other studies support a decrease in hair loss with androgenic alopecia. Hopefully, larger studies can help us learn more about the potential of this intervention and help clarify any areas of concern.

My Story

During the course of writing this book over the past three years, I started experiencing significant issues with alopecia areata, one of the most enigmatic hair conditions still challenging experts today. It was like the universe was challenging me to walk my talk or live my truth. Until that point in time, back in 2015, when I woke up one morning with a smooth, round, hairless area the size of a fifty cent coin on the back of my head, one of the things I knew for sure was that I had hair. It may have been greying, thinning, or perhaps even a little damaged, but these were all things for which I had solutions.

At first, my truth was to tell no one and cover it as much as possible. As you can imagine, this caused me great stress. The more I stressed, the more hair I lost. Soon, I had another area larger than the first now making its way to the front of my scalp. That's when I came to the conclusion that what I was doing wasn't working. I had to face my biggest fear, a fear so big that it prevented me, a physician, from seeking help from anyone. So I confronted it head on. I asked myself what was my biggest fear? My answer: fear of losing all my hair. Question: that would mean what? I would be bald. Question: that would mean what? I am no longer attractive. Question: that would mean what? It would mean that I am, somehow, less than. Wow, here I was, a physician, a mother, a small business owner, an author, a wife, and I was attaching my strength, my accomplishments, and my fierceness to my hair.

Life had unearthed one of my deeply hidden fears and reflected it back with the force of a megaton flood light. It was in that moment of realization that I found acceptance. In that moment, I recognized that it wasn't my hair or lack of hair that determined who I was or how I was perceived. I determined that. The way I felt about myself determined that. My hair was an opportunity for me to be creative and expressive about who I am and what part of my heritage, personality, journey, and message I wanted to share that day. With that realization, I finally exhaled. Now I was free to focus on finding solutions in whatever form they presented themselves.

Solutions presented themselves slowly and over time. My first decision was to push the reset button on my hair. I stopped using chemical straighteners on my hair, and I started to work on figuring out what my hair and scalp needed to be healthy. I also had to figure out what I needed to be healthy. I knew that as an autoimmune condition, alopecia areata could be exacerbated by severe stress. I then delved into what I do best, researching the

science and the studies. I looked at everything I could find, no

matter how small or seemingly insignificant. I asked myself the

same question over and over again, did the proposed mechanism of

action make sense? Was I able to follow the logic or the science?

After all my research, I created protocol for me that, so far, have

proven to be helpful. My protocol included injections of platelet rich

plasma (PRP) and stem cells into the affected areas, daily use of

curcumin, active B-complex and omega 3s. I have been following

this protocol since then, minus the injections, and have been able to

sustain continued progress. I also work diligently on trying to

manage my response to stressful events.

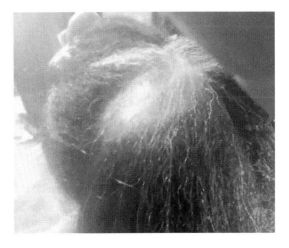

Figure 1: April 2016

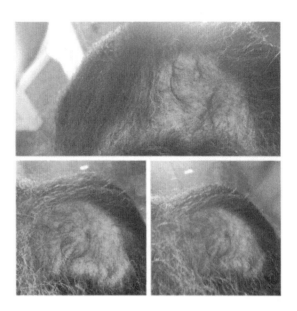

*Figure 2: two different areas being affected
Some regrowth noted after first treatment*

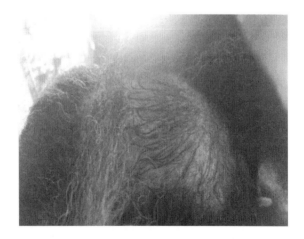

*Figure 3: steady growth with more follicles
Being involved, August 2016*

My Personal Routine to Keep My Hair Happy

My personal routine is still a work in progress. Like most women in their forties and fifties, I have experienced issues with keeping my hair in tip-top condition and, at times, it seems, issues with keeping the hair that I have on my head. I confess I have done my share of processing, blow-drying, flat-ironing, and even coloring. After all, I do possess a set of XX chromosomes.

My first bout of excessive hair loss came after the birth of my first child. Looking back, I see now that it was not only hormonal changes to blame but also the crazy diet I followed in an attempt to lose the weight I gained with my pregnancy. Remember, I wasn't born a holistic physician. I was born human. I did not experience as much hair loss with the birth of my second child as my eating habits were somewhat better. However, in my early to mid-forties, life with my hair became challenging. A new state, new climate, new hairdresser, and most importantly, years of hair abuse were catching up with me. I was experiencing increased breakage and hair loss and thinning. I knew I had to find a solution that would work for me.

I know many would say, at this point, that it was my hormones, but I believe imbalanced hormones are oftentimes just another casualty of an imbalanced life. After taking an honest look at my choices and patterns, from diet to hair products, I came up with a protocol for me. My first step was to take over my own hair care. I did this for many different reasons:

- It gave me leeway to try different products to determine their effectiveness for my hair type.

- I wanted to avoid excessively processing or chemically treating my hair.

- The thought of spending three to four hours at a time at the beauty salon just on my hair was beginning to overwhelm me.

Then I started the following protocol:

- I avoid harsh shampoos. In fact, I stopped using traditional shampoos altogether. I currently use nonsuds cleansers, such as Wen products. When I feel the need to shampoo, I use sulfate-free baby shampoo about once a month. This has significantly reduced the drying out of my hair and the subsequent breakage.

- I deep-condition weekly with an olive oil–based hair mask, keeping it on from fifteen to forty-five minutes with a heated towel wrap.

- I use a heat-protective product when I do blow-dry my hair to offer it some protection from the heat.

- I use topical melatonin around my hairline and have noticed a decrease in thinning.

- I sleep on silk or satin pillowcases.

- I reduced the amount of processing to my hair by covering grays with hair powder.

- When I feel tension all the way up to my scalp, I give in and schedule a neck and shoulder massage.

- I eat like my hair depends on it because it does. I consume healthy fats to keep inflammation down, lots of vegetables and fruits to fight free radicals and oxidation and to provide essential minerals, and finally, lean proteins to provide essential nutrients to the hair shaft.

Hopefully, by now, you can see that simply treating your hair from the outside isn't enough to ensure a healthy, full "garden." Instead, we must look deeper within to what we eat, drink, and even how we work and handle stress to ensure that our hair is the healthiest, and sexiest, it can be.

Creating Your Own Regimen for Healthy Hair

Creating your own hair regimen begins with embracing the history of the hair you were born with and interweaving it with the story of the hair you have currently. Perhaps your hair tells the story of your own strength and courage as a survivor. Maybe your hair reflects your journey to self-acceptance after years of being conditioned to believe that there is only one standard of beauty and self-expression. Whatever your hair's story, your goal is to nourish it, embrace it, and treat it with love. Doing so may finally allow you to connect with the goddess warrior within who knows that she is strong, sexy, and healthy regardless of where she is in her hair's journey. So whether you have long and thick hair, short and thinning hair, curly hair with a mind of its own, no hair at all, or

148

anything in between, choose to wear it with confidence. After all, it is not the style, the color, the extensions, or the wig that make you who you are; these are simply tools to accessorize your confidence.

To start creating your own healthy-hair regimen, I suggest taking inventory of the current health of your hair. I have listed a few categories below. If you check even one in the main category and over three in the additional category, it might be time for a hair makeover. Once you have established that you may need a hair intervention, proceed to the next section to help guide you through coming up with a plan of action to keep your hair as healthy as possible.

Category I	**Category II**
Main issues: The presence of any one of these issues requires a medical assessment.	**Additional issues:** The presence of more than three of these may require lifestyle assessment.
Excessive shedding of the hair	I process my hair once a month or more—this could be relaxing, perming, or coloring.

Areas of thinning hair	I apply heat to my hair daily or several times a week.
Areas of no hair	My scalp is oftentimes dry and flaky.
Excessive breaking of hair	I wash my hair daily.
Hair loss with weight gain and/or skin or nail changes	My diet consists of eating on the run, daily sodas, and less than seven servings of fruits and vegetables daily.
Hair loss on the body or face	I smoke.
Hair loss accompanied by weight loss and fatigue	My stress levels are extremely high.
Hair loss with osteopenia or osteoporosis	I have, or I am going through, menopause.
Have or am going through menopause	My hair appears dull and lifeless.

Your Healthy Hair Eating Plan

Your diet affects every part of your health and includes the health of your hair. For example, lack of zinc and good fats can lead to dry, flaky, and itchy scalp. Also, remember that the hair needs antioxidants and B vitamins for healthy follicles and, thereby, healthy growth. The good news is that the foods that nourish the hair also enhance the health of other parts of the body, such as the heart and the brain. See the following table to get an idea if you are on the right track.

Foods to include	Foods to limit
Omega-3 essential fatty acids: salmon, tuna, sardines almonds, walnuts flaxseed, chia seeds	Deep-fried foods Trans fats
Lean proteins: fish, poultry, eggs, meat	Processed meats
Antioxidants: vitamins E, A, and C; berries; green leafy vegetables; broccoli; Brussels sprouts; asparagus; carrots; red peppers; summer and winter squash	Canned and dried fruits (they often contain added sugars)
Foods high in iron and zinc: oysters, spinach, lentils, chickpeas, pumpkin seeds, liver, molasses, chocolate	To help limit risk factors for other health concerns, limit red meat to once a week.

Hair loss

If you are experiencing excessive hair loss or shedding, first rule out a medical condition that can be treated easily. Visit your doctor or your dermatologist for an evaluation to help determine the type of hair loss you may be experiencing. After taking a comprehensive history, including all the medications you may be taking, your doctor may order some of the following lab tests:

- TSH, free T4, free T3, and thyroid peroxidase antibody to evaluate the function of your thyroid
- Ferritin, total iron, hemoglobin levels to evaluate for iron deficiency
- Zinc RBC or alkaline phosphatase to evaluate for zinc deficiency
- Calcium levels and parathyroid hormone levels to evaluate for function of parathyroid glands
- Vitamin B_{12} and folic acid levels to evaluate for deficiency
- Testosterone, estrogen, and insulin to evaluate if your hormones may be playing a role in your issues with hair loss

Your doctor may also look at your hair strands under a microscope to help determine at what stage of the hair cycle you are experiencing the most hair loss. This can help him or her determine the most effective treatment. Sometimes, if the picture is still confusing, the decision may be made to perform a small scalp biopsy to determine the type of underlying inflammation.

If an underlying deficiency or condition is identified, then that deficiency or condition needs to be corrected. If it is determined to be an infection, such as a fungal infection, then an antifungal is usually prescribed. If an inflammatory condition is identified, then treatment is directed at reducing the inflammation. In autoimmune conditions, such as alopecia areata, oftentimes it is initially treated with a steroid injection directly into the affected area. Other people have experienced good results with stem cell injections with platelet-rich plasma into the affected area. You and your physician can determine the best course of action for you.

If your hair loss is hormonally related, then topical monoxidil with light therapy may help to stimulate the hair follicles to some degree. Some individuals have also found that hormonal-replacement therapy may help to stabilize excessive hair loss.

Taking Care of Hair from the Outside

If you came back with a clean bill of health from your physician, then your issue may be stemming from your haircare routine. For example, pulling the hair too tightly on a consistent basis can lead to hair loss from compromised blood flow to the hair follicles. Another possibility to consider is that you may have sensitivity to some of the ingredients in your haircare products that may be causing your scalp to become irritated. Scalp irritation potentially can impair the growth of healthy hair. Some potentially irritating ingredients are mineral oil and parabens.

Consider

If you are considering trying products with less potential irritants, a study published in the *Archives of Dermatology* in November 1998 showed promise in hair regrowth in individuals suffering with alopecia areata with a mixture of the essential oils thyme, rosemary, lavender, and cedarwood in the carrier oils jojoba and grapeseed oil. The researchers separated the patients into two groups. One group used this essential-oil mixture—two drops of thyme vulgaris, three drops of rosemary essential oil, three drops of lavender essential oil, and two drops of cedarwood essential oil mixed in three cubic centimeters of jojoba oil with twenty cubic centimeters of grapeseed oil—and the second group used the carrier without the presence of the essential oils. They were instructed to massage oil into the scalp for two minutes every night and then apply a warm towel to help with absorption of the oil into the scalp.

The results were very encouraging. Forty-four percent of the people in the group using the essential oils experienced some hair regrowth, compared to only 15 percent in the group using only the carrier oil. This is comparable or better to other treatments currently being used and carries no concerns about toxicity.

In another study, published in the journal of *Toxicology Research* in 2014, researchers sought to identify the way essential oils may have the ability to assist in the regrowth of hair. Using animal studies, they compared the effect on hair growth of peppermint essential oil, minoxidil (the FDA-approved hair-regrowth treatment), jojoba oil, and saline. The animal skin treated with topical 3 percent peppermint essential oil showed an increase in the amount of hair follicles, the depth of the hair follicles, and an increase in alkaline phosphatase and insulin growth factor in the hair follicle, both associated with healthy hair growth. The bottom line is that essential peppermint oil put more hair follicles in the anagen or growth phase, resulting in the faster regrowth of hair.

Love the Hair You're With

When you have done all you can, let go, and start loving the hair that you have now, and then let the real you shine through. Take this opportunity to color outside the lines because who drew those lines anyway? This is when the real fun can begin.

When you accept yourself and your right to fully express all the facets of your personality, then you can love and support each other without judgment. So, if see your fellow woman deciding to rock a bold bald look or braids or an afro or red hair down to her knees, you can say with a smile, "You go, girl. I see your spirit, I see your beauty, and I see your strength because I see the same in me."

Sexercise:

A "Sexy Back" Activity

We have all experienced "bad hair days," but don't let your hair determine how you feel; decide how you feel and let your hair be a reflection of that.

Today I feel:

- _____

_____

_____

_____

_____

_____

_____

Chapter 4:

Sexy Eyes–Let Your Sexy Shine Through

Can you remember the last time you really stopped to look carefully at your eyes? Not just to apply mascara or plump your lashes in the morning before work or at night before a big date, but really gazed into your very own eyes? I'm here to tell you that your eyes are one of your sexiest features, regardless of their size, shape, or even color.

Remember the eyes—the windows to the soul, and according to many forms of medicine practiced throughout the world, the doors to your health. In fact, there is even a specialty known as iridology that diagnoses primarily through the evaluation of the irises of the eyes. While I am certainly no iridology expert, western medicine also uses the eyes to peek into the health of the rest of the body. Did you know that, oftentimes, the eyes can reflect the health of the liver, the brain, and perhaps even the heart? It gives us a heads up that blood sugar levels may be too high or blood vessels may not be as healthy as we would like them to be. If our blood vessels are damaged, as in conditions such as peripheral vascular disease (PVD) or diabetes, then our ability to have a healthy sexual relationship may be compromised.

Not yet convinced of the power of the eyes? Did you know that scientists can determine if you are attracted to someone simply by looking at the degree of dilation of your pupils? In fact, this is apparently an ancient secret. In Italy, in the sixteenth century (okay, not so ancient), women would use belladonna eye drops to dilate their pupils because they felt it made them more appealing. Now, we may not have to go this far to get our sexy back (after all, belladonna is toxic), but we can start taking steps to maximize the health and sexiness of our eyes.

Basic Structures of the Eye: Seeing is Believing

The eye consists of a complex series of lenses, cones, nerve cells, and blood vessels that communicate so seamlessly with the brain that their efforts in helping us navigate and appreciate the complex beauty that is life oftentimes goes unnoticed. Since this is not an ophthalmology textbook, the goal here is to understand the basic concepts about how we see, so that it might make it easier for you to recognize when there is something amiss.

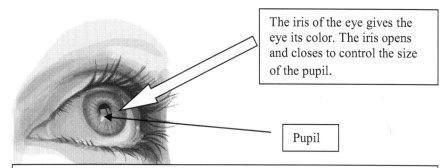

The iris of the eye gives the eye its color. The iris opens and closes to control the size of the pupil.

Pupil

The cornea is the transparent outer layer that covers the eye. Light is refracted through the cornea, and then passes through the pupil to enter the eye.

So, how does the eye work? If we were to simplify, we can imagine the eyes work similarly to a camera. When we are looking at an object, we are actually seeing light that has reflected off the object, entering the eye through the cornea. The cornea then refracts the light and passes it through the pupil. The light then enters the lens of the eye, which changes shape to focus the light unto the structure in the back of the eye called the retina. The lens of the eye is surrounded by tiny muscle fibers called ciliary muscles. These muscles contract and relax, changing the shape of the lens, allowing us to see both near and far. When the muscles relax, the lens flattens, giving us clearer distance vision. When they contract, the lens assumes a more curved shape, allowing us to focus on objects that are closer to us.

The retina is a very thin layer of nerves comprised of structures called cones and rods because they are shaped like cones and rods. Cones are roughly located in the center of the retina in a structure called the macula. From this location, and in the presence of bright light, cones allow us to see images in front of us in bright color and in sharp detail. Rods are located in the periphery of the retina outside the macular. When the rods are functioning normally, they allow us to see in dim light, help us to detect motion, and enhance our peripheral vision. When light hits the light sensitive nerves of the retina, the light signal is converted to an electrical signal, which is then transmitted to the brain for interpretation. The brain takes these impulses and translates them into an image, thus completing the miracle that is vision.

There have a multitude of books written to help us navigate the latest makeup tips to help make our eyes pop or lashes appear longer or create eyes that smolder. While I too am grateful for these tips, imagine if we apply these tips to healthy eyes; that's taking sexy up several notches!

Healthy eyes are sexy eyes because when your eyes are healthy, they:

- **Look better;**

- **Feel better;**

- **Perform better;**

- **Last longer;**

- **Require fewer accessories.**

Tips for Healthier Eyes: *Protection is Prevention*

The first step to maintaining healthier eyes is to protect them against the damaging effects of the elements, much as you would protect your skin. Remember, protection is the first form of prevention.

We are aware that prolonged exposure to UV radiation from the sun not only increases our risk of skin cancers, but also contributes significantly to premature aging and wrinkling of the skin. If this is true for the skin, imagine the damage that prolonged exposure to sun can cause to the sensitive eye tissues. It is estimated that about 99 percent of the UV radiation that enters the eye is absorbed by the anterior structures of the eye. That would mean significant exposure to the two major refractive surfaces of the eye, the cornea and the lens. Ultraviolet radiation can lead to damage to the cornea, which can leave the eyes feeling constantly sandy or gritty.

The conjunctiva, the outermost layer of the eye, is also very susceptible to damage from UV radiation. The conjunctiva plays an important role in keeping the eyes clear and free of debris such as dust, wind, dirt, etc. Prolonged exposure to UV radiation can cause discoloration of the conjunctiva that leaves it looking muddy, dull, and discolored. It can also contribute toward the excessive growth of eye tissues producing a structure called a pterygium that can, over time, grow over the lens and obstruct vision. UV damage to the eyes can leave us looking older and more tired than we feel.

While many of us are aware that UV damage can come from unprotected, excessive exposure to the sun, we also must be aware that tanning beds can also produce these damaging wavelengths.

One of the simplest, most practical, affordable, and convenient ways to protect your eyes from the sun and wind is to wear sunglasses that offer the full array of UV (UVA and UVB) protection. So, get in the habit of wearing sunglasses anytime you're outdoors. If you enjoy biking, walking/running, skiing, or otherwise are involved in an outdoor activity, consider wearing goggles to protect your eyes or wraparound glasses to prevent sand, wind, and dirt from invading and possibly abrading the eye surface, or conjunctiva. Wearing a broad-brimmed hat, especially during those long, hot summer days, also can help to keep those damaging rays from making direct contact with these windows to our souls.

A diet high in astaxanthin, lutein, zeaxanthin, and other carotenoids have also been shown to offer some protection against UV damage of the eyes. This is in no way a substitute for wearing your sunglasses and hats, but it doesn't hurt to have additional protection. Numerous research studies have shown astaxanthin to be a powerful antioxidant that offers some protection against free radical damage caused by UV damage. In fact, it is estimated that it is sixty times more powerful as an antioxidant than vitamin C, and I love vitamin C.

What is astaxanthin? Astaxanthin is produced by the microalgae *Haematococcus pluvialis* to protect itself from the UV waves when water evaporates. Part of its mechanism of action is that it seems to have the ability to directly absorb some of UVB rays before they can do damage to the eye tissue. A good source of astaxanthin is wild-caught salmon. Other brightly colored vegetables and fruits high in carotenoids may offer additional eye protection, as well. This is another notch in the belt of eating healthy.

"Monitor" the Amount of Computer Glare per Day

It can be a challenge to reduce the amount of time we spend on computers because of how ever-present they have become at work, at home, and in life in general. After all, I am currently writing this chapter parked in front of a computer. From working at a computer eight hours per day to staring at a tablet or TV for fun or gaming to texting nonstop, we can spend the majority of our day staring at screens of various brightness, sizes, and glare. But studies show that long stretches of time spent staring at a computer screen can lead to big trouble later on, particularly for our eyes. In fact, the phrase Computer Vision Syndrome has been coined to reflect the constellation of symptoms that may occur from extended overuse of the computer or other electronic devices with reflective screens.

While it is currently thought that exposure to electronic and computer glare does not cause permanent damage, "Computer Vision Syndrome" can lead to:

- **Headaches;**
- **Neck and shoulder pain;**
- **Double or blurred vision;**
- **Tearing;**
- **Difficulty focusing;**
- **Burning sensation, and even**

169

- **Fatigue of the eye muscles and**

- **Dry Eyes—not enough tear production.**

There are several ways to reduce computer glare. For example, reducing the amount of light in your office or computer workstation can help reduce reflective glare. Experiment with your computer and/or monitor placement until whatever form of light you prefer no longer provides as much, if any, computer monitor glare. There are also special filters, or screens, you can buy to cut down on glare.

Another suggestion is to position your computer in a way that minimizes eyestrain. Some suggestions for optimal screen placement are:

- Place the top of the screen at eye level;

- Tilt the screen back ten to fifteen degrees;

- Position the computer twenty to thirty inches away from you.

In addition to cutting down glare, I recommend monitoring the amount of time you spend at any one screen. Our eyes need rest, just like the rest of our bodies. So if you work at a computer all day, take a break from the screen every two hours or look away from the screen every twenty minutes for twenty seconds focusing on a point twenty feet away. Get up and move around, get a drink of water, go to the bathroom, or look at a book or piece of paper that may need your attention, if only to give your eyes a rest from computer overload. Blinking frequently may also help lubricate the eyes with your tears.

One of the simplest ways to prevent a host of eye problems—strain, soreness, and particularly, dryness—is simply to keep our eyes moist and lubricated with a variety of over the counter drops and lubricants now available on the market today. Moist eyes are healthy eyes, particularly as we age, and in addition to looking better, clearer, and healthier, they will feel better. If you are experiencing significant dryness, a persistent gritty feeling, pain, or change in vision, a visit to your eye doctor would be in order.

Eye Care for Life

The American Optometric Association, or AOA, recommends that individuals between the ages of eighteen to sixty should get their eyes checked every one or two years. If you're over the age of sixty, then annual eye exams are recommended. Patients who are considered at risk by their eye doctors, meaning they have a pre-existing eye condition, wear contacts, have had eye surgery, suffer from diabetes or hypertension, or have a family history of eye problems, should consult their physician for how often to schedule an appointment.

While going into detailed eye pathology is well beyond the scope of this book, my goal is to provide you with basic information of some of the most common chronic eye pathologies that can compromise the health and vitality of your eyes. From allergies to diabetic retinopathy, your eyes can tell the story of you.

During the eye exam, your eye doctor will not only be assessing your vision, but also the health of the structures that are immediately visible to the naked eye and the structures in the back of the eye that require special instruments to visualize. He will be able to tell if your eyes have been excessively exposed to the sun, show signs that allergies are responsible for the puffiness and redness, if your vision problems are caused by changes associated with aging (presbyopia), cataracts, or something more sinister such

172

as macular degeneration or glaucoma. He or she can see signs of diabetes, high blood pressure, or high cholesterol reflected in the back of the eye. Below is a description of three relatively common eye conditions your eye doctor will be looking for when he or she examines your eyes. While this certainly does not encompass all the intricacies of the eye exam or all possible eye conditions, my hope is that it starts giving you some understanding of how your eye works.

Glaucoma

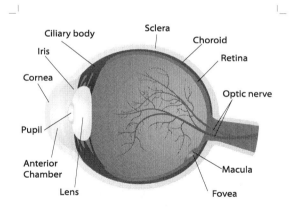

Glaucoma is an eye condition that can cause blindness if left untreated. There is a fluid that circulates in the very front chamber of the eye (anterior chamber) that nourishes and moisturizes the tissues it comes in contact with, keeping them healthy. Usually, this fluid flows freely into and out of the anterior chamber. Like a clogged drain, if this fluid drains too slowly or not at all, then pressure can build up inside the eye. This pressure can then increase to a point where it crushes the nerve in the back of the eye (optic nerve) that helps you see.

This optic nerve connects the eye to the brain, and if this nerve is damaged, then the connection to the brain is lost, and you will no longer be able to see. Your ophthalmologist (eye doctor) can recognize this condition early and begin treatment to reduce pressure, thus preserving vision.

While this book is not about glaucoma, I hope it stresses the importance of regular eye exams so that eye pressure can be monitored by your eye doctor. An immediate visit to the eye doctor or the emergency department is indicated for sudden changes in vision and/or eye pain.

Cataracts

Cataracts affect the lens of the eye. The lens of the eye is usually clear, and like any other lens, if they become cloudy, then it becomes difficult to see through them. A clear lens allows light to pass through to the back of the eye, focusing images so that they are clear and crisp. Cataracts are basically proteins that slowly accumulate in the lens, causing a cloudiness that prevents light from shining through effectively. Cataracts are painless and tend to develop slowly over time; thus, they initially may not be noticeable. However, the foggier the lens become, the more difficult it becomes to see clearly.

While the biggest risk factor for developing cataracts is age, diseases such as diabetes and chronic use of certain medications, such as steroids and diuretics, can increase the risk of developing cataracts prematurely. In fact, diabetes is the leading cause of blindness in the US. At times, diabetics can develop intermittent blurriness in vision because the lens of the eye swells when blood sugar gets too high.

Other conditions that increase the risk of cataracts are exposure to UV radiation (sunlight), ionizing radiation (flying), trauma to the eye, cigarettes, and heavy alcohol consumption. Here again, we see how lifestyle choices can have an impact on health. As an aside, babies can be born with cataracts. This is referred to as congenital cataracts.

Is it possible to prevent cataracts? First, to begin to answer that question, we must first look at some mechanism of cataract formation. One mechanism of cataract formation is excessive accumulation of blood sugar or glucose in the lens of the eye. Diabetics are particularly prone to this form of cataract formation. When glucose builds up in the lens of the eye, it is acted upon by an enzyme called aldose reductase to form an alcohol sugar called sorbitol. High concentrations of sorbitol in the lens cause an osmotic effect, thus drawing an excessive amount of fluid into the lens causing it to swell. This can then lead to damage of the proteins in the lens, leading to the formation of cataracts.

Several studies suggest that the topical use of a medication that inhibits the activity of aldose reductase can help to reduce the formation of cataracts formed by this polyol pathway. With this being said, it is worth noting that there are several foods that seem to have some aldose reductase activity. What are these magical foods? Good news, they are foods we all have access to and should be included as part of a healthy lifestyle as they have other potential benefits, as well. Some of these are spinach, lemon, cinnamon, basil leaves, pomegranate, apples, oranges, and black pepper.

Macular degeneration

Macular degeneration is one of the leading causes of blindness in people over the age of sixty. The macular is the small area located in the back of the eye that is responsible for the clarity, color, and detail we are able to see in the center of our vision. It is also a part of the retina, the nerve tissue that lines the inside of the eye that detects and transmits light to the brain (see diagram above).

When the macula becomes damaged, you can lose central vision, not see as clearly, or perceive colors as well, and even have blind spots in your vision. Risk factors for developing macular degeneration are age, hereditary, smoking, high blood pressure, obesity, high cholesterol, and light skin color. While age and genetics are out of your control, paying attention to lifestyle again may help impact this disease. Discussion of the forms of macular degeneration is beyond the scope of this book but suffice it to say, early detection of this condition can lead to treatment that can slow the progression of this disease and preserve vision.

Presbyopia

As we get older, the eyes lose the ability to focus on close objects; this condition is referred to as presbyopia. It generally starts around the age of forty. It is not considered a disease but rather a normal part of the aging process. As we age, the lens (see above diagram) of the eye becomes less flexible, thus losing some of its ability to focus. Some signs of presbyopia are:

- Arms not being long enough as you have to hold reading material further away from you in order to focus;
- Headaches and eye fatigue when reading;
- Words now seem blurry at normal distances, or you wish everyone would stop printing words smaller and smaller.

Can anything be done about presbyopia, short of stopping or reversing the aging process? Most individuals resort to reading glasses that help them see close up. There is the possibility of fitting one eye with contact lenses that help you see close up or a procedure called conductive keratoplasty that uses low level radio frequency to correct near vision in one eye while leaving the other eye untreated to see distances. I recommend discussing these options with your ophthalmologist to determine which one, if any, would be right for you.

What about using eye exercises to improve presbyopia? In my opinion, this would be challenging to do since it would require these exercises to improve the flexibility of the lens. I am also not aware of any studies that show significant improvement in vision with this method.

What about pinhole glasses? For those of us who are not familiar with pinhole glasses, they are glasses that look like sunglasses but the lenses are replaced with lenses that have multiple, small pin-sized holes. Focusing through these holes can correct the refractive issues that come with presbyopia, thus allowing you to "read the fine print." These glasses are not practical for long-term wear as they do not allow you to see much else.

Dry Eye Syndrome

The eyes depend on tear production to keep them moist and lubricated. Tears are made up of water, oils, mucous, electrolytes, and antibodies, all designed to protect the eyes and enhance vision. The mucous layer is produced by glands lining upper and lower lids called meibomian glands. The lacrimal gland produces the tears that lubricate the eyes. The tears then drain into the lacrimal canal to the sac and empty into the nasolacrimal duct. Healthy eyes are protected and covered with a thin layer of tears at all times, referred to as a tear film. A decrease in tear production, and/or conditions that dry out the tear film lubricating the eyes, can lead to dry eye syndrome.

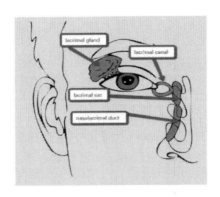

Some conditions that can dry out eyes are a dry environment, such as air conditioning and heating systems; prolonged exposure to wind, sun, and high altitudes; and staring for long periods of time that causes one to decrease blinking frequency. Conditions that do not allow the eyelids to close properly, such as Bell's palsy, menopause, getting older, and the use of certain medications, such as antihistamines and decongestions, can also cause this syndrome. A deficiency in vitamin A can also increase the risk of developing dry eyes. Certain diseases such as diabetes and autoimmune diseases, such as lupus, Sjogrens's, and rheumatoid arthritis, can also decrease tear production, thus predisposing one to dry eye syndrome. Excessive alcohol use has also been shown to exacerbate dry eye symptoms.

Some signs and symptoms of dry eye syndrome are:

- A constant, sandy, gritty feeling in the eye or feeling like there is something in the eye;
- Sensitivity to light;
- Burning sensation;
- Redness;

- Itching;

- Blurred vision;

- Quick onset of eye fatigue after reading for a short period of time;

- And a feeling of dryness in the eyes.

If you are experiencing persistent issues with any of the symptoms above, then a visit to your eye doctor is in order. There are now multiple treatments available for dry eye syndrome that can help alleviate your symptoms and avoid the potential damage that can be caused by persistent loss of the protective moisture barrier of the eye.

Lifestyle for Healthy, Sexy Eyes

Now that we have an idea of how your eyes work, let's examine how lifestyle and environment impacts the eyes and its many structures.

Smoking and the eyes:

Smoking increases your risk of forming cataracts and developing macular degeneration. In cataract formation, it is believed that smoking directly damages the cells of the lens of the eye, thus leading to premature clouding of the lens. Also, cigarettes contain the heavy metal cadmium, along with many other toxic substances. Some researchers believe that smoking causes cadmium and other heavy metals to concentrate in the eye, thus creating the opacity associated with cataracts.

Smoking increases the risk of developing macular degeneration by as much as four times. It is thought that apart from directly damaging the macula, cigarette smoke also causes damage to the blood vessels that supply the retina (see diagram above).

Smoking can contribute to other eye conditions, such as dry eyes. The good news is that research shows that if you stopped smoking now, you can reduce your risk of developing macular degeneration by up to 7 percent in one year and up to 12 percent in five years. That is amazing in such a short space of time. Smoking also damages the collagen in the skin, thus leaving the skin under the eyes saggy and loose. This is definitely not sexy and confidence boosting.

UV Rays and the Eyes

UV from sunlight and tanning beds can damage the lens of the eye, thus increasing the risk of cataracts. Are you aware that it is estimated 22 million Americans suffer from cataracts? Knowing that cataracts can significantly impair vision, this is certainly an incentive to protect those valuable peepers.

UV radiation can also cause damage to the surface of the eye, causing the growth of a benign tissue structure called a pterygium. This is important because, apart from being possibly unsightly, this tissue can grow over the cornea of the eye, potentially obscuring vision (see figure below).

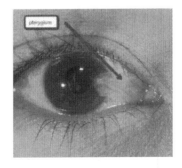

Once this vexing tissue has formed, the only treatment for removal is a surgical approach. The problem is that even with successful surgical removal, there is a significant risk that this problem can recur. Recently, however, there has been a new exciting development. It seems that an old drug used to thin the blood called dipyridamole, when applied in eye drop form, has demonstrated success in dissolving this tissue. This treatment is not currently approved because more testing needs to be done, but this is certainly exciting news for those suffering with this condition.

Another harmful byproduct of exposure to UV rays is painful sunburn to the cornea of the eye referred to as snow blindness (photokeratitis). Snow blindness interferes with vision, causing one's vision to appear spotty like falling snow, hence the name.

As you can begin to see, chronic and even short-term exposure to UV radiation can cause significant damage to the eye. So, wear broad-spectrum UV wraparound sunglasses to provide your eyes with the maximal protection. To dispel a myth, cloudy days have just as much UV exposure as bright sunny days as UV light can easily penetrate any cloud cover.

I am sure that many of you have heard of the UV index. This is a scale developed by the EPA as a way of relaying the amount of UV exposure we are exposed to each day. The scale goes from 1 to 11 with 1 being lowest exposure and 11 being extremely high exposure.

UV Scale	Interpretation
<2	low
3-5	moderate
6-7	high
8-10	Very high
>11	Extremely high

Nutrients for Healthy Eyes

What you eat unequivocally impacts the health of your eyes. Interestingly enough, the nutrients that benefit your brain and heart also benefit the eyes. A diet high in good fats, such as omega-3s and antioxidants from deeply colored fruits and vegetables, can protect the eyes from damaging UV light and help preserve your vision. Other nutrients shown to protect eye health are vitamin C, vitamin E, and of course, lutein and zeaxanthin. So what foods are good for your eyes? Below is a list of foods to eat regularly to keep your eyes vibrant and functioning optimally.

Foods	Nutrients
Strawberries, Oranges, Green peppers, Grapefruit	Vitamin C
Wheat germ, Sunflower seeds, Almonds, Avocado, Olives	Vitamin E
Broccoli, Kale, Spinach, Grapes	Antioxidants, Lutein, and Zeaxanthin

Pumpkin seeds, Oysters, Turkey	Zinc
Salmon, Sardines, Herring	Omega-3
Pumpkins, Squash, Carrots, Sweet potatoes	Beta-carotene

Vitamin C and Eye Protection

According to the American Optometric Association, vitamin C reduces the occurrence of cataracts by as much as 67 percent. The research suggests that a minimum daily intake of 300 mg is needed to be effective in preventing the formation of certain types of cataracts. Of note, there are many fruits and vegetables high in vitamin C, such as strawberries, oranges, and beets that can provide a healthy dosage of vitamin C daily.

Vitamin C, in combination with other nutrients such as beta-carotene, lutein, zinc, and vitamin E, has been shown to reduce or slow down the rate of deterioration of macular degeneration. What do most of the above nutrients have in common? You guessed it—they are great antioxidants, especially in combination as one is often used to rejuvenate the other. Some also have pigments that are able to absorb some of the harmful UV rays.

The researchers at Oregon Health & Science University found that for the retina (the nerve cells lining the back of the eye) to function normally, it must be saturated in a bath of vitamin C. If we recall, the retina helps us with sharpness, acuity, and color of an image. The fact that vitamin C is needed for retinal cells to function normally points to the potential role of this vitamin in helping us see more clearly.

N-Acetyl Carnosine and the Eye

Carnosine is a small peptide or protein building block. Unlike vitamin C, it can be made naturally in the body and is found in high concentrations in the heart and skeletal muscles. Research suggests that the use of carnosine in the form N-acetyl carnosine applied topically to the eyes in drops can reduce the risk of the formation of cataracts. Carnosine is not only a powerful antioxidant but has also been shown to prevent the damage that occurs when a sugar molecule attaches itself to protein or fat cells, a process called glycation. Glycation causes damage when it attaches to these cells. In the case of cataracts, this causes damaged protein to accumulate in the lens of the eye, causing the clouding associated with this condition. Carnosine may be able to prevent this from occurring.

N-acetylcysteine (NAC) and the Eye

N-Acetyl cysteine is an amino acid that is an extremely powerful antioxidant. It has the ability to increase the production of our body's levels of its own antioxidant called glutathione. Several animal studies suggest NAC can prolong the lifecycle of the light sensitive nerve cells in the back of the eyes called the retina. This has the potential to impact the occurrence of macular degeneration. One form of NAC, called N-acetylcysteine amide (NACA), seems to be more effective as it can penetrate cellular membranes to work at deeper levels inside the cells. With this special property, NACA seems to be able to reduce the occurrence of cataracts, as well.

Lutein and Zeaxanthin and the Eye

Lutein and zeaxanthin are two powerful antioxidants that are found in very high levels in the eye, especially in the structures mentioned earlier, the lens, the retina, and the macula. One of the functions of these pigmented antioxidants is to absorb the damaging UV light before they can penetrate and wreak havoc with your vision and eye health. In fact, one large study found that the combination of these nutrients with other antioxidants, such as vitamin E and zinc, was able to slow the progress of age related macular degeneration, thus preserving vision for a longer period of time.

So where in the world do we find such powerful nutrients? You guessed it—vegetables such as spinach, kale, and broccoli contain high levels of these antioxidants.

So how do you know if you have sufficient lutein and zeaxanthin in your vital eye structures, such as the macula? The good news is your eye physician now has the ability to measure these levels in the eye with a test called macular pigment optical density. This test measures the density or the thickness of these pigments in the macula. Research with this tool found that a higher density correlated with decreased risk of developing macular degeneration and better vision. *This is yet another reason to have regular and truly preventative eye exams.*

Hope for the Future?

As of this writing, science is still searching for effective ways to prevent the progression of eye conditions that can rob us of the precious gift that is our sight. For conditions such age related macular degeneration the prognosis can be quite grim. Stem cells may offer some hope to those who have already experienced the ravishes of retinal degenerative conditions such as age related macular degeneration (ARMD). Researchers have been able to create retinal cells from mesenchymal stem cells (MSC) and implant created cells into the retina of the affected eye. These transplanted cells seemed to offer protection against further degeneration of the retinal cells.

One animal study using retinitis pigmentosa (a genetic disease that causes blindness) as the model for retinal degeneration demonstrated some preservation of vision and retinal function with the use of mesenchymal stem cells transplanted via intravenous infusion.

Research is just beginning to scratch the surface of the potential of mesenchymal stem cells to be a part of the solution to many conditions that threatened our health today. While scientists are busy doing their part, let us continue to do our part to preserve and protect the precious gift of sight.

Healthy, Sexy Eyelashes

If given a choice between healthy, lush-appearing eyelashes and brittle, thinning eyelashes, most individuals will opt for the former. I would imagine that is why the sales of mascara and other products designed to make eyelashes appear longer and thicker remain quite robust. While I confess to being part of that billion dollar sales boom, I believe that applying mascara to healthy lashes gives a far more dramatic effect than using mascara to try to make unhealthy lashes look healthier.

So how do you keep your lashes in tip top shape? Eyelashes follow a similar growth pattern to any other hair on the body; they have a growth phase (anagen), a resting phase (catagen), and a falling out phase (telogen). So anything that impacts the hair on your head could also impact the growth of your eyelashes.

The growth and health of the eyelashes also very much depends on the health of the eyelids. In fact, conditions such as blepharitis or inflammation of the eyelids can trigger eyelashes to go into the telogen phase and fall out prematurely, causing eyelashes to appear thin and brittle.

So part of maintaining healthy eyelashes, is practicing good eyelid hygiene. This includes removing all eye makeup before going to bed, tossing eye makeup that is over a month old, and avoiding the practice of sharing personal products, such as mascara or eyeliner.

What about products that claim to grow eyelashes, do they to work? By now, I am sure that many of you are familiar with the story of Latisse. Once upon time, the medication in Latisse, bimatoprost, was used as eye drops to treat individuals with glaucoma. Lo and behold, some of these individuals started growing longer and thicker eyelashes. What if we could make this side effect into the main attraction, thought the powers that be? Bingo, Latisse was born.

Latisse is now FDA approved for hypotrichosis (sparse growth) of the eyelashes and seems to work quite well in many individuals. A common side effect, noted by many individuals, is burning and irritation of the eyes. It is also possible, according to the literature that accompanies Latisse, for it to darken the color of the eyes in some people. This, however, seems to be a rare occurrence.

What if you are, somehow, being challenged with an illness or a condition that does not allow you to grow eyelashes or leaves your eyelashes looking thin and sparse? Or, what if genetically your eyelashes are naturally thin or fair? My opinion is that health is not measured by the length or the thickness of your eyelashes; that may be one way you choose to express yourself in that moment or that day.

My Healthy Eyes Routine

I admit to taking my eyes for granted in my younger years. I very seldom wore sunglasses, never gave a thought as to how my diet was affecting my eyes, and thought that perfect vision was something that was guaranteed to me for life. Now, in my fifties, when the letters on the "small print" are not as crisp as they use to be and my eyes get irritated at the end of the day due to the demands placed on them during the day, I remind myself not to sit around and lament about what I "should" have done. Instead, I remind myself of the words my mother would say: "When you know better, you do better." So now, I have developed a routine to take care of the precious gift of sight that I have been given.

My first line of defense is to visit my Ophthalmologist annually. Yes, I spend the rest of the day not being able to see anything, but it is a small price to pay to identify early signs of trouble. I ensure that I protect my eyes from the damaging UV radiation of the sun by wearing UV protection sunglasses. There are so many sizes, shapes, and colors that sunglasses can become a fun personality statement, not just something you "have" to do. I remove all eye makeup before going to bed. This keeps my eyes from being irritated and red in the morning; not to mention, it prevents the clogging of the oil producing glands along the lash line.

To further nourish and protect my eyes, I work on incorporating foods high in lutein as frequently as possible. I also, oftentimes, take an additional lutein, bilberry, and zeaxanthin supplement as I find that they reduce my sensitivity to glare. Finally, I work on keeping my eyes moisturized with lubricating drops in combination with an antioxidant eye drop that soothes my dry eye symptoms from being in front of the computer too long.

Developing Your Own Healthy Eyes Routine:

Maybe you already have your own healthy eyes routine in place, if so, great! However, if you are just starting the process, you can look at the following checklist and try to identify potential areas of concern for you. Oftentimes, the best place to start is with a visit to your eye physician.

Check to the left to mark the true statement

	Lifestyle		Nutrition		Protective Habits
	I exercise regularly		I eat a variety of leafy, green vegetables		I wear sunglasses
	I don't smoke		I eat a variety of brightly colored vegetables		I pay attention to the amount of time I spend on the computer
	I limit my alcohol intake		I eat deeply colored fruits, such as blueberries and bilberries		I schedule my annual visit with my eye doctor
	I exercise regularly		I eat foods high in omega, such as sardines and tuna		

Look at the areas that are lacking a check and work on those areas

Finally

When you have ensured that your eyes are the best they can be, have some fun playing up your eyes. If it is okay with your ophthalmologist, and you are in the mood to just change your look a little bit, try some colored contacts. If that does not appeal to you, then try the newest makeup trends, such as the smoky eye or the nude eye. If playing with makeup is not your style, then try having fun with your sunglasses. Try different styles and shapes. Want to be just a tad extra (to quote my daughter), go to the store, try them on, and take a bunch of selfies. Let's stop judging each other and ourselves about our style preferences or how we choose to express ourselves that day or that week. There are many nuances that make you who you are; feeling free to express them is part of being sexy.

Parting Words about Sexier Eyes

Your eyes perhaps really are the windows to your soul. They can give others a glimpse into who you are and what you are feeling without you having to utter a word. They can encourage, beckon, show kindness, or they can glare with disapproval. They can radiate confidence and health, or they can reflect to others the uncertainty we feel about ourselves. So whether your eyes reflect the blueness of the sky, or draw people in because they radiate the warmth of molten chocolate, or burn with the intensity of the deepest charcoal, it is important to keep them in the best condition possible. Healthy eyes have an almost luminous quality, a way of drawing people in and making them more curious about you. That is sexy!

Chapter 5:

Love the Skin You're In

"It's not what you look at that matters, it's what you see."

–Anonymous

When we look at ourselves in the mirror or in pictures, we all want to look as if we are carrying our own internal filter. We want that glow that says we are healthy, happy, and sexy. Sometimes, we might be so focused on the laugh lines around our eyes or the frown line between our brows that we may completely miss the story of our skin. The skin can tell a story of health, a story of joy, confidence, and sometimes, even a story of our pain. I believe that, many times, what we are earnestly searching for when we study our reflection in the mirror are signs that say I have faced life's challenges, and in the end, I chose confidence, I chose strength, and I chose me.

When I look at women like Helen Murin and Jane Fonda, I find myself being drawn in by their seemingly effortless beauty and sex appeal. Yes, they have great bone structure and perhaps the best makeup artist in the world, but I have come to realize that what shines through is confidence, self-acceptance, and the choice to value and take care of one's self in the face of a society that often tries to devalue individuals as they get older. That, in my opinion, is sex appeal of the highest tier. It reinforces, for me, that being healthy and confident and choosing to continue to love, contribute, dream, and live life unapologetically is the foundation of getting your sexy back. Everything else is a form of self- expression.

The Basics or the Boring Stuff

For those of you who have read my first book, some of this will be review. For those of you who haven't, you won't need to do so, this stands on its own. The following is a statement that you have probably read, in one form or another, multiple times before. The skin is the largest organ of the body and is our first line of defense against the environment. However, are you aware that at the same time our skin is protecting us against the environment, it is also busy interacting with our environment to provide us with essential nutrients such as vitamin D, and it also helps us regulate our body temperature? It is packed with immune cells to help us fight off infections and transmits information about our environment to the brain through our sense of touch.

It is also often one of the first organs to start showing little telltale signs of aging and, most importantly, our health. We are often judged to be healthy, ill, tired, happy, or even sad based on the condition of our skin. Also, we often judge ourselves based on what we see in the mirror. What we might overlook, is the health of our skin, is as much an inside job as it is an outside job.

Structural Integrity of the skin:

Our skin is made up of three primary layers: the epidermis, dermis, and the hypodermis. The epidermis is the top layer of the skin. It is waterproof and helps retain moisture in the skin. This layer of skin also contains cells that are part of the skin's immune system. Other cells in this layer, called melanocytes, produce the melanin responsible for pigmentation of skin and filtering harmful ultraviolet radiation from sunlight. As you can see, this is quite a busy layer.

The dermis is the second layer of skin and is made up of a thick layer of fibrous and elastic tissue that is approximately 80 percent collagen. It helps the skin maintain its elasticity, strength, and smoothness. Elastin is another protein present in the dermis and helps provide elasticity to the skin through its interaction with collagen. The dermis also contains nerve endings, some hair follicles, oil secreting glands (sebaceous), and blood vessels. The dermis also supplies nourishment to the epidermis.

There is a layer under the skin known as the subcutaneous layer. This layer contains adipose tissue (fat), sweat glands, and blood vessels. It forms a cushion underneath the skin that prevents it from falling onto the bone. All three layers work together to give our skin a smooth, youthful appearance.

Also present in the skin are substances known as GAGS (Glycosaminoglycans) and proteoglycans. These are specialized sugars with the ability to hold many times their actual weight in water. GAGS help the skin seal in moisture and appear plump and well nourished. I am sure you may have heard of one of the most famous GAG, hyaluronic acid. This compound can hold many times its weight in water. By attracting and holding on to water, hyaluronic acid helps the skin appear plump and resilient. Due to this unique ability, hyaluronic acid is used in some of the most popular facial fillers such as Restylane and Juvederm.

Basic Aging of the Skin

Visible aging of the skin can start as early as age 25. These changes begin to accelerate in our 40s, when hormonal changes and decreasing hormonal levels begin to play a significant role. The skin can be affected by many factors including aging, environmental changes, poor nutrition, medications, stress, and hereditary factors. As we get older, the skin cells divide slower, and the top layer of skin gets 10 percent thinner every ten years. The number of melanin cells in the top layer shrinks. This causes the skin to appear thinner and more translucent. Another noticeable change is the formation of excessive pigmented areas known as age or liver spots in the epidermis layer. This is usually secondary to damage from excessive sun exposure.

Changes are also taking place in the dermis. The blood vessels in the dermis become more fragile and rupture easily causing skin bruises. This, along with thinning of the skin, could worsen the appearance of those dreaded under eye circles that make us look tired and older than we really are. The oil producing glands become less active. The amount of moisture holding GAGS in the skin decreases leaving the skin drier, looser, and less plump.

Environmental conditions like excessive sun exposure, poor nutrition, and smoking can speed up the loss of collagen and elastin and accelerate the aging process (Photochem Photobiol, 1993 Dec;58(6):841-4.). UVA radiation in sunlight weakens collagen and causes the excessive production of abnormal elastin. This abnormal elastin is not able to maintain the function and structure of native elastin, thus causing the skin to appear less firm.

The exposure to free radicals, generated by smoking and excessive sun exposure, causes a decrease in collagen production and also activates the production of an enzyme known as metalloproteinase. This enzyme breaks down damaged collagen in preparation for removal and remodeling. Also, much of the new collagen being produced is abnormal and does not possess the tensile strength and elasticity of the original level. To add insult to injury, the fatty subcutaneous layer, the hypodermis, also thins out and makes the skin appear looser.

All of the above combined with the effects of gravity, poor lifestyle choices, and habitual facial expressions can leave our skin with distinct wrinkle patterns (crow's feet or laugh lines), loose sagging skin, loss of facial volume, dry, uneven skin tone, hyperpigmentation, and broken capillaries.

Now that we have a very basic understanding of what happens to the skin as we age, it's time to create the story of your skin. If you look in the mirror and love your healthy glow and those tiny laugh lines simply accentuate the joy reflected in your face, then you are there, relish it, embrace it, and share it. However, if what you see reflected back is not the story that represents who you are now or speaks of your current journey, then perhaps the story of your skin may need some editing. Perhaps it is time to start exploring the many options that science, research, and nature have provided us to help enhance and reflect the inner fire and glow that we want to start speaking for us before we even say a word. We can then simply decide to love the skin we are in because it tells the story of us perfectly.

We are bombarded on a daily basis with lotions and potions that claim to not only stop the aging process but also to magically return our skin to the look of our youth. Oftentimes, the image used to convey this message is one of a beautiful young woman in her early twenties. Your skin today is not the same as it was when you were younger, but it is no less important, beautiful, or vibrant. For example, my twenty-year-old self cannot tell my story today. That would be fiction and not fact. Focusing time, resources, and energy trying to recapture something that has passed leaves very little to create the now. Also, the message that goes along with that is one of not being enough where you are now, and that is not empowering. If you do not feel empowered, that is often reflected in the quality of your skin. You want your skin to reflect health, passion, and confidence in who you are now.

What Damages the Skin?

We are a product of what we eat, how we think, and the environment in which we live, and our skin also reflects these truths. Intuitively, it makes sense that our skin, the largest organ in the body and, oftentimes, the first organ to interact with our environment, can be significantly impacted by the harshness of the elements. What we may not stop to consider is the impact of other lifestyle habits on the health and integrity of our skin. For example, can our food choices, activity, and stress levels contribute to premature aging of the skin? According to science and just plain old observation, the answer is a resounding yes! This is good news because it lets us know that we are not completely at the mercy of our genetics; we are able to take steps to protect our skin and help it deflect some of the ravishes of time.

Environment and the Skin:

- **Sun and UV Radiation:** As mentioned previously, prolonged exposure to UV radiation from the sun can compromise the integrity of the skin by weakening one of the main components that gives skin its firmness and resilience, namely collagen. The end result is that the skin is now more prone to premature wrinkles, loss of volume, and increased sagging.

UV radiation can also cause such damage to the DNA of skin cells that hinders their ability to repair and replicate normally, thus leaving them more susceptible to cancerous mutations. In simple terms, excessive exposure to the sun increases your risk of developing cancerous lesions on the skin. Other conditions such as hyperpigmentation, sunspots, and uneven skin tone can all be exacerbated by prolonged exposure to the powerful rays of the sun.

- **Air Pollution:** The increase in air pollution from industrialization has been linked to an increase in inflammatory skin conditions, including premature aging of the skin. The increased ozone in the air decreases the antioxidant levels in the skin thus leading to being more susceptible to environmental damage.

- **Menopause:** This is one you can't control that can bring with it a significant change in the internal environment to which your cells are exposed. There are several hormones that contribute to the health and well-being of the skin including estrogen, testosterone, progesterone, and cortisol.

  In postmenopausal women, decreased estrogen content in the skin has been associated with decreased production of collagen, increased thinning, and increased propensity for dryness and wrinkling of the skin. High levels of cortisol have been known to cause excessive thinning and increased fragility of the skin. Menopause may not directly impact the levels of cortisol, but the increased levels of stress and inflammation that frequently accompanies getting older can potentially adversely impact the levels of cortisol, thus having an indirect impact on the condition of the skin.

Lifestyle Habits and the Skin:

- **Smoking and the Skin:** At this point in time, I am sure that there isn't anyone on the face of the planet that has not at

211

least heard about the pitfalls of smoking. We know that it increases the risk of many cancers, heart disease, and even strokes, but did you know that it can make your skin act and look much older than it is? As mentioned above, it has been demonstrated in the lab that smoking hinders the production of normal collagen. Smoking also causes direct DNA damage in the skin, much like prolonged exposure to UV radiation, thus potentially increasing risk of skin cancers, as well.

- **Lack of Exercise**: According to the University of Illinois, consistent, moderate exercise can help decrease inflammation, thus helping the skin heal faster. Speaking of exercise, one study published in *JAMA Dermatology* 2018, found that thirty minutes every other day of specific facial muscle exercises helped participant look up to 2 to 3 years younger. If you don't think this is a big deal, I ask you to look at a picture of yourself three years ago and compare it to an image of you now, and see if you notice any changes.

Sometimes, you will be amazed by the difference a few years can make.

Since loss of facial volume is one of the major components that can make a face appear older, it would seem reasonable that firming up the muscles can help replace some of that volume loss. Clearly, the drawback to this practice is that the exercises would have to be done consistently to help maintain the results.

- **Nutrient poor diet-** A diet that is poor in antioxidants, vitamin C, zinc, essential fatty acids, and essential amino acids can potentially lead to less than optimal condition of the skin. A diet high in refined carbohydrates and sugars can increase the risk of developing diabetes. If proteins in the body are chronically exposed to excessive sugars, as found in uncontrolled diabetes, then those proteins can be irreparably damaged. Studies show that in diabetes, collagen, the protein that helps to keep the skin looking firm and healthy, is damaged at an accelerated rate, thus leading to premature aging of the skin.

- **Increased Stress levels:** Have you ever paid attention to your facial expressions when you are worried or extremely focused? More often than not, the most common expression will be a frown. Facial expressions are frequently habitual. Creating tension or creases in the same area over and over again will eventually lead to the formation of a line or wrinkle in that area. Now you know why the lines between the eyes are called frown lines.

  Stress can impact the skin so much more than the mechanical creation of frown lines. For example, excessive exposure to cortisol and adrenaline, two of the body's stress hormones, can also have a negative impact on the skin. Cortisol in persistently high quantities can cause thinning and easy bruising of the skin while contributing to loss of muscle mass and tone. Adrenaline causes the blood vessels in the skin to clamp down, thus decreasing blood flow to the skin and its vital structures. This could potentially lead to the skin being continually deprived of the nourishment it needs to thrive and maintain its healthy glow.

Signs Your Skin May be Damaged:

As we get older, our skin is exposed to more and more environmental and other physical insults that may cause the skin to age prematurely or exhibit other signs of unrelenting damage to the skin.

- **Age spots or liver spots:** Whatever name you use, we are all familiar with the sound patches of hyperpigmentation that appears in certain individuals in areas that have been chronically exposed to the unrelenting UV radiation emitted by the sun. So, common places that age spots would occur are the back of the hands, face, and shoulders, all areas that usually have the most sun exposure.

  Even though these coalescent areas of hyperpigmented lesions can appear unsightly, age spots are benign and do not need to be treated. If desired, these spots can be addressed with agents such as kojic acid that are designed to fade dark spots. The best way to treat age spots is to develop routines that decrease your exposure to prolonged sun exposure. For example, the diligent use of

215

sunscreen and clothes with UV protection factor of fifty or above can help to keep these spots at bay. If you have age spots and you notice a change in color or character, then visit your dermatologist immediately for a thorough skin evaluation.

- **Fine lines and wrinkles:** Premature lines and wrinkles may also be an indicator of excessive damage to the skin. If we recall from previous discussion, prolonged exposure to UV radiation, smoking, and even excessive pollution in the air can affect collagen and moisture production in the skin, thus leading to premature formation of lines and wrinkles.

- **Loss of volume and sagging skin:** Volume loss can occur not only from loss of the structural integrity of the skin but by also bone and muscle loss, as well. As we get older, we begin to lose bone mass, and that includes the bones of the face that provide the scaffolding for the shape and contour of the face. As you can imagine, if the support that keeps everything lifted and firm begins to sag, then what follows is a gradual downward movement of the facial structures.

Common areas that are impacted by volume loss are the lines between the nose and lips (nasolabial line) and the area directly beneath the corner of the lips (marionette lines).

Some individuals feel that the appearance of these lines can leave them looking more tired and sad than they actually feel. This can sometimes impact the way that they perceive themselves or amplify their concerns about how others view them. Sometimes, in our zest to express concern about others, we oftentimes comment on how sad or tired they look today, and we frequently follow that by asking if they are okay. Imagine if you heard that phrase even two or three times a week. How would that make you feel?

Having said that, are there viable solutions available to help address some of these concerns? We have already mentioned the use of minimally invasive substances, such as hyaluronic acid, that are used to restore volume and structure to the face temporally. For those of us who simple do not like needles, we mentioned the use of ultrasound directed heat using devices such as Ulthera to stimulate collagen production with the goal of gradual subtle lifting of the skin.

Healing and Rejuvenating the Skin: Steps to Maintaining Healthy Skin

- Dermatology visit

- Sunscreen

- Nutrition

VITAMIN C

Vitamin C is necessary for the formation of collagen in the tissues. Humans lack the ability to produce vitamin C naturally in the body and must obtained it through foods. Research has shown that oral vitamin C supplementation does not increase the concentration of this important vitamin. However, studies show that topical application of vitamin C is one of the most effective ways to boost collagen formation in the skin.

Vitamin C is also a potent antioxidant that helps neutralize free radicals in the skin. Free radicals are unstable, reactive molecules that form during the body's normal metabolic reactions. They need to bind to another molecule to stabilize. When free radicals bind to collagen, they form breaks in the collagen molecule that change the chemical structure and cause it to become more disorganized. This new form of collagen loses its tensile strength and, thus, makes the skin look saggy and wrinkly.

Several studies have shown that vitamin C can reduce the appearance of fine lines and wrinkles in as little as twelve weeks! Not only did they see improvements in fine lines but skin also showed improvement in skin tone and clarity. Believe it or not, even acne and age spots also diminished significantly. Below is a list of benefits that demonstrates why topical Vitamin C is a crucial part of my daily regimen:

- It moisturizes
- Encourages growth of collagen
- Softens
- Exfoliates and cleanses
- Helps diminish the appearance of fine lines and wrinkles

- Improves skin tone and clarity to give you that glow that you thought you may never see again

RETINOIDS

Retinoids are a group of active ingredients derived from vitamin A. There are a number of different types of retinoids found in skin care products including retinyl palmitate, retinol, and tretinoin (retinoic acid). Retinoic acid is the active form of vitamin A derivatives, and other forms including retinol and retinyl palmitate must be converted to retinoic acid before they can deliver any beneficial effects to the skin. Retinoic acid is the form found in prescription vitamin A creams.

Retin A has been shown to increase cellular turnover in the top layer of skin making skin appear brighter and smoother. In sun-damaged skin, collagen formation is decreased. Retinoic acid can boost the production of collagen by up to 80 percent and help restore some of the smoothness and plumpness to the skin. This form of vitamin A also has been shown to improve the appearance of hyperpigmented lesions, such as liver spots and melasma.

Well, this sounded so promising that a group of researchers, much like myself (curious), wondered what would happen if they combined retinol and vitamin C as a treatment in postmenopausal women. They found that this combination was able to partially reverse, yes reverse, the skin changes that occur with chronological aging and the signs of skin damage that occur with prolonged exposure to the damaging UV rays of the sun. Helping my skin remember what it did when it was younger is one reason that retinol is also part of my daily routine.

NIACINAMIDE

NIACINAMIDE, a derivative of Vitamin B3 (niacin) has shown in several studies to offer anti-aging benefits when applied topically to the skin. Topical niacinamide has the potential to reduce the appearance of fine lines and wrinkles, reduce hyperpigmentation spots, and return some of the youthful glow to the skin. It has also been shown to improve the hydration of skin and conditions such as rosacea—another notch in your arsenal belt.

PEPTIDES

A peptide is formed when several amino acids are linked. Some peptides are believed to stimulate the formation of collagen and decrease the activity of enzymes that destroy elastin. This action helps the skin hold some of its resilience. One such peptide is palmitoyl pentapeptide. In test tube studies, this peptide was found to stimulate the formation of collagen, elastin, and GAGS, all the things that help the skin maintain characteristics of younger looking skin.

Other peptides, known as neuropeptides, have shown in laboratory results to block the release of neurotransmitters from the nerve to the muscle. One hexapeptide is called Argireline. In theory, this peptide would be able to stop contractions of the muscle, revealing a more relaxed look, similar to the actions of botulism toxin A. While results may not be as dramatic as botulism toxin A, one study showed a 30 percent reduction in the depth of wrinkles, and 30 percent sure trumps zero percent. Another positive, no needles required.

Hyaluronic acid

This is another favorite of mine and certainly has been garnering a lot of media and cosmetic attention. For those of you who are familiar with facial fillers and injectables you are probably aware that one class of fillers is hyaluronic acid based. Because this substance can hold many times its weight in water, it is a perfect substance to fill out the hollowing in the facial features that some of us experience during the aging process. But can applying this substance topically offer any potential benefits? After all, injectables are not for everyone.

As mentioned above, hyaluronic acid is found abundantly in younger skin. It helps plump skin and keeps it looking dewy and fresh. As we get older, the skin drastically loses the ability to produce and retain this substance. This could be due in part to the decline in estrogen that accompanies the aging process. The *American Journal of Dermatology* 2012 reminds us that estrogen helps maintain hyaluronic acid and other GAGS in the skin and also helps maintain barrier function. The result is plumper, more resilient skin.

As we get older, the skin becomes thinner and, therefore, no longer holds on to moisture as efficiently as it once did. We may then be left with dull, dry skin that looks much older than it should. Imagine if we can get this miracle substance to absorb into the skin with just topical application—game changer, right? Well, consider the game changed because topical application of hyaluronic acid does provide some skin benefits and has been shown to get absorbed by the skin. In fact, pharmaceutical companies are taking advantage of the skin permeability of hyaluronic acid to deliver medications deeper into the skin to treat certain skin conditions such as actinic keratosis.

What about wrinkles you may be asking? Good question. Think about this—where is the skin the thinnest, the most fragile, and therefore, more prone to developing over-exaggerated lines and wrinkles? You guessed it, around the eyes. If you have very expressive eyes and love to laugh out loud and smile frequently and your skin is thin, dry, and low on elastin, then you may be prone to more of these expression lines around the eyes.

Now, remember, this is about you being fabulously flawed, so if you feel every single one of those lines were earned, and they remind you of the life of joy you have lived and continue to live, then be and embrace that fully. If, on the other hand, you know that you are fabulous but you would like the lines to be softer to highlight the sparkle in your eyes even more, then feel free to do that, as well. Remember, we are here to represent that we are all fabulous and unique and special regardless of how we choose to express that.

Enough of my soap box, back to hyaluronic acid. Yes, say researchers, hyaluronic acid can significantly improve skin hydration and elasticity, and this can lead to decreases in the depth and appearance of those lines and wrinkles around the eyes. Here is the part to pay special attention to—they got significantly better results with low molecular weight hyaluronic acid. Caveat, not all hyaluronic acid are created equal.

Alpha Hydroxy Acids (AHA)

These are chemicals that have the ability to improve skin texture and reduce the appearance of fine lines by encouraging the shedding of the outer layer of the epidermis or upper layer of skin. This allows for better absorption of products into skin while brightening its appearance. It is also thought that they can stimulate some minimum collagen production. Examples of these chemical exfoliators are:

- Lactic acid—It is said that Cleopatra took baths in soured milk to help keep her skin smooth and beautiful. Little did she know that she was setting a trend for future generations. Lactic acid is an acid derived from the fermentation of milk. It comes in different strengths, most of which are now available over the counter. It is considered one of the milder alpha hydroxyl acids. What's it good for: Helping you get your glow on. It helps replenish the skin barrier to hydrate dry skin. One of my trade secrets is that I use it every day to keep my skin from flaking and drying out.

- Glycolic acid—Glycolic acid is derived from plants with high sugar content, plants such as beets and sugar cane.

Considered a little more irritating than lactic acid, this power house also comes in different strengths. The milder versions are available over the counter while the more concentrated forms can be obtained through your dermatologist or skin care specialist. Other plant extracts, such as papaya, are also used as gentle exfoliators.

- This is not meant to be an all-inclusive list of chemical peels and exfoliators, but they are certainly two of the most common.

Antioxidants: Taking UV Protection to the Next Level

There is one statement that generally I feel confident making—preventing damage is usually always easier than attempting to repair it. That, my friends, is the secret to an antioxidant's role in helping the skin age gracefully.

- **Green tea extract**, the new sunscreen? Now before we go ditching our favorite sun protection, let us understand how green tea can contribute to the healthy aging of your skin. It might be a little bit more complicated than brewing some tea and washing your face or as simple as tea bags on the eyes. Where is the science? Well, there are several studies that show that the application to the skin of several extracts of green tea prior to UV exposure (simulated sunlight) protected the skin in several ways: First, the extracts reduced the number of cells that suffered sunburn and protected the cells in the skin from UV damage. Secondly, and a great bonus, is green tea extracts reduced the DNA damage that can be created after exposure to UV radiation. One can see how this can lead to much less photoaging of the skin, or as we like to call it, sun spots or age spots.

- **Vitamin E**: Definitely a friend to the skin. Did you know that the top layer of your skin contains a significantly high level of vitamin E in the form of alpha tocopherol? Another marvel of this amazing skin that we take for granted every day. A lipid or fat soluble antioxidant in high concentrations at the top layer of the skin not only protects the skin from the elements but also serves to prevent the loss of moisture from the skin.

- **Ferulic acid**: more than an antioxidant but a stabilizer. Above, we discussed and sang the praises of Vitamin E and Vitamin C. Even though these vitamins have been proven effective time and time again, the major issue has been the stability of these vitamins on exposure to air and the environment. This is important because you need to understand that just because a formulation reads that it contains vitamin C does not mean that this formulation is capable of providing the benefits noted in the studies. If we were able to find a way to protect these age fighters, then they can have maximum impact on those lines and wrinkles.

  Well, enter Ferulic acid to do just that. Ferulic acid is a potent antioxidant found in seeds such as apple, coffee, and flax. It is also found in the cells of other plants, as well. Researchers found that when ferulic was combined with vitamin C and vitamin E, there was a significant improvement in the performance of either of these vitamins, along, or even in combination, with each other. Their ability to reduce the signs of aging in the skin and protect against oxidative damage doubled. Moral of the story, on your way to reversing the signs of aging, you must think about preventing further damage if your skin routine is to be complete.

- **Marine Algae**: To algae or not to algae, that is the question. If you have ever gone on a quest to find the perfect antiaging solution for your skin, I am sure you have come across red algae or some other form of algae being touted as the next miracle in skin care. But is this science fact or fiction?

Now the name marine algae is a dead giveaway that lets you in on the secret that these algae have been sourced from the sea. What is so special about algae? You guessed it; they contain special polyphenol antioxidants referred to as phlorotannins. The magic seems to lie in their ability to inhibit the enzyme tyrosinase that cause the over deposition of melanin, thus potentially making it an effective ingredient to prevent photo aging or darkening of the skin from exposure to the sun. It also protects against UVA and UVB radiation that we are exposed to on a daily basis just by walking outside. Remember, this radiation has the potential to damage DNA in the skin cells, and damaged DNA is oftentimes a precursor to the development of malignancies.

Red microalgae seem to have anti-inflammatory properties derived from a polysaccharide-type chemical that they contain. Topical application of the extract from the algae decreases inflammation not only by inhibiting the movement of leukocytes, or white cells in the area of irritation, but also stopped these immune cells from sticking to the lining of the tiny blood vessels supplying the skin, thus preventing a forest fire of inflammation. One can expect that conditions such as eczema could potentially benefit from the particular algae.

There are many species of algae, and each seems to contain its own version of photo protective chemicals. Learning all the names and properties are well beyond the scope of this book.

- **Ceramides**: ceramides are a heterogeneous group of lipid or fat molecules that are found in high concentration in the layer in between the cells called the stratum corneum. This fatty layer also contains a specific ration of free fatty acids, ceramides, and cholesterol that join together to form a protective barrier in the skin that helps to hold on to moisture, thus keeping the skin hydrated and protected from the elements. Loss of ceramides in the top layer of the skin can lead to dry, flaky, itchy, skin conditions such as eczema and also cause the skin to lose the plump, rosy appearance of hydration.

Out of the Box Thinking: You want me to do what?

Sometimes, it seems that we dare to try anything in the name of beautiful skin. Here are some that I am sure you have heard about. Let me know after reading about it if you are going to swipe right or left on these purported beauty treatments:

- **Leeches**—well, in the olden days, as the story so often begins, leeches were a medicinal wonder and used for about whatever ailed you. The idea was that the leeches would suck the evil spirit, bad blood, and poisons out of the body, therefore resulting in a miraculous cure. That, however, very seldom panned out the way it was intended. After more than a few poor outcomes, the use of leeches in medicine fell out of favor. Enter the twentieth century and leeches came back with a vengeance. This time as a way to improve circulation in wound healing or post surgically. Leeches have chemicals in their saliva that helps thin the blood, therefore allowing blood to reach the areas of concern more easily.

So how did these vampires of the water turn into the latest beauty treatment? Enter leech facials. This is a procedure where leeches are either placed on the face or some other part of the body to collect your blood. The blood is then extracted from the leeches and smeared onto the face as a treatment mask. The idea is that the chemicals in the leeches' saliva would allow the nutrients and growth factors in the blood to penetrate further into the skin, thus delivering therapeutic benefits deeper into the skin while increasing circulation to the skin. Bingo, the results, smoother, firmer skin, right?

In my opinion, based on the information available right now, I am going to say that this one is not ready for prime time. Apart from the obvious concerns about any procedure that involves the use of blood borne products, there is not enough data to support that this form of therapy is any more effective than a hydrating mask and may be fraught with slightly more complications.

- **Low level infrared light**—Therapy or just shining a red light on your face?

Light therapy is another therapy that has been used throughout history to treat various ailments from moods to acne, and now, it has entered into the regenerative arena with the promise of giving you younger, smoother skin with no downtime. Certainly an attractive idea, but is there science behind the conjecture?

Several small studies using a variety of different wavelengths of light ranging from 633nm, 830 nm, to 1130 nm have reported some positive results. In the experimental Petri dish, it seems that low-level laser therapy has the ability to stimulate the growth of fibroblasts, the cells that promote healing and structure.

Now, is there a magical wavelength that seems to be the most effective? How long do the effects last? How many treatments are necessary? These are all questions that require further investigation. This might be one of those that you would categorize as worth a shot, doesn't hurt, and I have disposable income.

- **Platelet Rich Plasma Injections or PRP**

What is PRP and how does it work? The answer is in the name. Platelets are specialized cells in the blood that produce and secrete specialized compounds referred to as growth factors. These growth factors do just that, they help cells repair and rejuvenate the way they did when you were younger. The idea is that injection of this specialized serum to the areas that need rejuvenation will help that tissue turn back the hands of time a little bit.

How is PRP collected? Here is the good news; it is prepared from your own blood; therefore, there is no risk of you acquiring blood borne disease from someone else's blood. The bad news is it does require the practitioner to draw your blood. So your feelings about needles may determine if this makes it to your to-do list. The blood is then spun in a specialized medical centrifuge to extract the platelets and the growth factors they produce.

How is it applied? The platelet rich plasma is injected the way Botox and fillers are injected. Maximal results are usually expected within four to eight weeks.

How does it work? Good question, and the jury is not completely in, but research is revealing several potential mechanisms of action. Most of the research right now is pointing to PRP being able to induce new collagen and fibroblast formation in the skin. If we recall from earlier, these structures go a long way in preventing the skin from sagging.

Are there other applications for PRP? PRP is currently being used for things like hair restoration, erectile dysfunction, and even joint pain from wear and tear. It is not currently approved by the FDA for these purposes as it is not a drug. But anecdotal reports would suggest that many people are getting good results.

Minimally Invasive Techniques

Now that you have colored outside the box, let's hop back inside and get an idea of some of the minimally invasive techniques that have been FDA cleared or approved for facial rejuvenation. This is simply a brief mention of what these techniques are and in no way is meant to be a comprehensive review. You will be able to access those through your dermatologist, plastic surgeon, or aesthetic physician's office, and there, you should be able to get all your detailed questions answered.

- **Laser resurfacing of the skin:** Lasers are loosely placed into two categories—ablative and non-ablative lasers. Ablative lasers refer to the fact that some of the top layer of skin is removed. This form of laser therapy penetrates more than the non-ablative form and may require sedation or injected pretreatment for pain. Due to the deeper nature of treatment, ablative lasers may require up to two to three weeks to fully heal.

By the opposite token, non-ablative lasers pass through the skin layers but do not remove any layers of the skin. This form of laser therapy can oftentimes be performed with topical or even no numbing medicine at all. There is usually minimal or no down time with this type of laser.

Regardless of the type of laser, it is recommended that you do not smoke for two weeks before and at least two weeks after procedure so that you can get the best results possible. Also, keep in mind that for optimal results you may require multiple treatments.

- **Ultrasound**: Focused ultrasound therapy is now being used to lift and firm the skin above the eyebrows, neck, and recently, the décolletage. One such FDA cleared device is called Ulthera. The idea is that focused ultrasound energy stimulates the body's own production of collagen. The results are gradual and the full effect is seen after two to three months. Many people opt to use this treatment for mild to moderate skin laxity.

This, and other non-invasive modalities, cannot give surgical results. Be honest with your doctor about your expectations so you can have the information to make the right decision for you. Keep in mind that as with all modalities, individual results will vary.

- **Fillers**: Fillers generally refer to a class of medical grade substances that are FDA approved to temporally restore volume to the face. Falling into this category are fillers composed of hyaluronic acid, such as Juvederm and Restylane, and the volume expander composed of calcium hydroxylapatite, such as is found in the brand name Radiesse. Both of these substances are naturally found in the body, so allergy testing is usually not indicated. The effects of these fillers can last anywhere from six months up to two years.

These fillers can come in different thickness and consistency based on the area of the face to be addressed. To find out what would work best for your concerns, I recommend booking a consultation with a qualified aesthetic physician such as a cosmetic surgeon, dermatologist, or other physicians with training in these techniques. Do your homework; after all, it is your face.

- **Botulism toxin**: Botox, or botulism toxin, is used in very controlled small dosages to relax the muscles around the eyes and the forehead that can contribute to premature wrinkling. Relaxation of these muscles can allow contralateral muscles to exert a lifting effect on the affected area. Botulism toxin is used to treat dynamic lines—those are lines that are formed by movement of the muscle in question. It most likely will not have an effect on lines that are significantly prominent when the face is at rest. It is important to acknowledge this to avoid unrealistic expectations and disappointment. In my opinion, the practitioner who uses botulism or substances like it should have an understanding of the dynamic push and pull of the musculature face to get the best results possible. Again, I can't stress this enough, do your homework. A medically qualified practitioner will use products FDA approved for wrinkle treatment. Not all botulism products are created equal. It is your health; do not risk it or discount it.

My facial routine:

Over the course of many years, I have found that I needed to change my facial routine every five years or so. As I have gotten older, I have discovered that indeed my skin has gotten drier, thinner, and has experienced some volume loss. I have found that the easiest way to begin to discover what works for my skin is to accept where it is now. If I constantly focused on what it was in my twenties, I would be missing out on major opportunities to provide my skin with the essentials that it needs to age well and with grace.

The first thing I discovered as I entered my fifties was that my skin was becoming drier, so my cleansing routine had to become milder. I found that cleansing my skin with a hydrating makeup wipe remover accomplished several task. First, it kept my skin from drying out by providing moisture from the beginning, so I didn't feel like I had to run to a moisturizer as soon as my face was clean. Second, it removed all of the makeup and dirt at the end of the day without having to wash my face multiple times, and third, it was super convenient. My favorite makeup remover wipe is Neutrogena hydrating wipes. For me, it works like no other, hydrating without leaving an oily film while removing all traces makeup.

The next thing I had to come to terms with is the inherent decrease in the cellular turnover rate of my skin that accompanied aging. My skin was starting to appear dull, lifeless, and tired. I was starting to also notice discolorations, minor acne from clogged pores, and the appearance of fine lines. At this point, I decided to introduce Retin A and vitamin C, though not together. Both of those ingredients are known for their ability to enhance collagen formation and increase the cellular turnover of the skin, thus creating the appearance of a smoother, firmer complexion with the return of a healthier glow. I use the Retin A product at night and the Vitamin C product in the morning. I found, this way, my skin tolerated both products without any issues.

Finally, I needed to address hydration and moisture retention. This I addressed with the addition of a hyaluronic acid product that contained ceramides. I use this twice a day to help my skin maintain that look of hydration. I top this off with sunscreen and sun protection in the day. These are my daily staples. I may add other products that contain other antiaging ingredients intermittently if I feel that my skin is being particularly challenged. For example, I use a hydrating toner that contains the antiaging ingredient, acetyl Hexapeptide-8.

Your Facial Routine:

Great, now you have all of this information, how do you put it all together in a way that makes sense for you? Perhaps the easiest approach might be to identify issues that you are currently experiencing so you can target the appropriate remedy. For example, if you feel that your skin is on the drier side, you may want to focus on ingredients that hydrate the skin. If you feel that your issue is lack of firmness and premature fine lines and wrinkles, you may want to focus not only on hydration but also ways to help the skin appear firmer and more resilient. If you know the only way you can be consistent with a facial routine is to keep it simple, then you look for products that do just that.

Below is a table to help you to determine where to start.

Habits		Concerns		Solutions
Smoker		Can lead to premature aging and wrinkling of the skin. Can also increase risk of skin cancer.		Stop smoking. Increase vitamin C rich foods. Start applying sunscreen. Visit your dermatologist for screening
Diet low in antioxidants and essential fatty acids		Can lead to premature aging and wrinkling of the skin		Increase the vegetables and fruits in your diet. Also, be sure to include foods high in omega 3 and

				other essential fatty acids
Does not wear sunscreen or sun protection		UV radiation damage to the skin creating accelerating aging. Increases risk of skin cancer as well		Avoid prolonged exposure to sunlight. Wear sunscreen. Use physical sunblock if sensitive skin or concerns
Aging skin— could start as early as 30 years of age		Part of aging process is loss of volume, bone and muscle loss, thinning of skin and decrease collagen, and other substances that help with		Address individual concerns. Mature skin tends to need moisture. Consider hyaluronic acid and ceramides. It may also need help with shedding top skin layer to reveal

		moisture retention	newer cells. Consider vitamin C. If skin can tolerate it, a retinoid product may help. Mature skin may also be more sensitive so pay attention to that as well
High pollution exposure		Can create concerns similar to smoking	More challenging to resolve as it often involves factors that are out of your control. Some things that you can try—house plants and antioxidant moisturizers

Complexion appearing dull		Can leave you looking tired and uninterested		Consider vitamin C and/or a glycolic acid cleansing pad followed by hydrating cream
Skin losing volume		Can lead to sagging and loss of contour		Products with DMAE may be helpful. May have to consider fillers or other minimally invasive procedures. Consult your aesthetic physician

Chapter 6:

Stop and Smell the Roses

When you own your breath, nobody can steal your peace. ~Author

Unknown

An iconic nose, what does that even mean? Am I talking about the chiseled nose of a Greek god or a nose that turns up perkily at the end? Absolutely not! In fact, I do not advocate any particular size, shape, or slope of the nose. The aesthetics of the nose is, as we know, based on cultural and individual preferences and has little to do with the function of the nose.

In my opinion, the sex appeal of the nose has more to do with its function and less to do with its appearance. What makes the nose incredible sexy is its ability to evoke nostalgia and memories from a simple whiff of a hauntingly familiar fragrance. For example, the way your husband's cologne makes your heart skip a beat because it reminds you of the first time you met or maybe the first time he said "I love you." Have you ever experienced pure bliss by inhaling a scent that transports you back to the idyllic week you spent sitting with your feet buried in the sand, listening to the waves as they pour onto the shores over and over again, creating the most soothing sound you have ever heard? If you have ever gotten dressed to go out on a date and reached for your favorite perfume because you knew when you applied it, you would go from feeling pretty good about the way you look to knowing you are certainly one of the sexiest women on the planet, then you have experienced the power of the nose.

In addition, your sense of smell can enhance one of our most sensuous experiences, the ability to taste. Have you ever tried eating your favorite warm, gooey chocolate chip cookie only to find that your sense of taste is so dulled by your stuffy nose that you might as well be biting into a piece of a cardboard box? If you have ever experienced biting into a plump, succulent strawberry and following it with a sparkling glass of your favorite champagne and inhaled the sensation of the sweet juices of the strawberry mixed with the tiny fireworks of bubbles, then you can begin to appreciate the value of your sense of smell.

Now, if we distinguish our sense of smell from breath, we have another wonderful feature of the nose—the place where peace can begin. With breath, we can inhale peace, life, and love. With breath, we can begin to center ourselves so that we can begin to notice our inner yearning to connect to our dreams and our passion. With breath, we can begin to inhale our deepest passions and desires and exhale the manifestations of those dreams.

As if that weren't enough, your nose is your first alert system in more ways than you can imagine. Oftentimes, we can smell danger well before we can visually identify the source of that danger. But, did you know that your nose can also be the first

249

subtle warning sign that all may not be well with the brain? In fact, recently using a ruler and peanut butter, researchers at the University of Florida were able to identify those individuals at risk for developing Alzheimer's disease. It seems that the sense of smell is affected in certain neurological disorders well before other changes can be clinically documented. A healthy nose can boost your spirits, help you breathe more easily, help you enter vixen mode, and more importantly, can be the first sign of dysfunction and imbalance in the body.

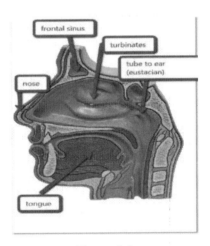

Figure 6-1

Function of the nose:

When you breathe in, the blood vessels underneath the surface of the nose and the small hairs in the nose warm, humidify, and filter the air that passes through on the way to the lungs. But, how does the nose smell? The act of smelling occurs in several steps.

First, anything that you are able to smell gives off molecules that then enter the nose and attach themselves to tiny hairs (cilia) located on some nerve cells in the nose. These nerve cells then transmit that information to the brain via the olfactory (smell) nerve. This nerve is one of a set of twelve nerves from the brain that sends and receives information from the structures in the head, allowing us to smell, taste, and see. Together, these nerves are referred to as the cranial nerves. The olfactory nerve is Cranial Nerve I.

It is estimated that humans are able to detect up to 10,000 smells! How does this ability to smell tap into our emotions, mood, and even memory? The olfactory nerve is located in a part of the brain that allows it to closely interact with the part of the brain commonly referred to as the "emotional brain." The emotional brain is associated with memories, emotions, and feelings. However, smells themselves do not create memories or feeling. This seems to be a learned response. When we first smell a certain scent, we may associate it with an event, person, or a place. The brain then creates a link between that scent and the memory or the feeling that accompanied it. For example, you may have associated the scent of lemons with the time that you and your best friend spent hours squeezing multiple lemons for your first lemonade stand. That may have been a really happy time for you, so now, whenever you smell lemons, you experience a lift in your moods without necessarily understanding why.

Marketers are pretty savvy to this phenomenon. Ever been into a model home and experience that homey, comfortable feeling? That may have something to do with the scent of baked goods emanating from the kitchen of that model home, tapping into that feeling you had when you baked chocolate chip cookies with your mom. Some studies suggest that this link between smell and emotion may start as early as being in the womb. For example, infants who were exposed to a lot of garlic while still in the womb showed a preference for the smell of garlic.

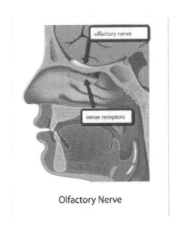

Olfactory Nerve

Frenemies of the Nose

If you are like most humans on the planet, you have experienced, at least once in your life, nasal congestion or stuffy nose to the point where it interfered with your ability to taste or smell. I am sure you can recall how miserable you felt during this time. For those of you suffering from nasal allergies, this may be something that you cope with on a seasonal, if not daily, basis. Besides allergies and infections, there are several other factors that may interfere with our sense of smell and, at times, even our ability to breathe efficiently through our nose. Besides anatomical obstructions like a deviated septum or abnormal growths, it seems that genetics may play a role, as well.

Scientists have discovered that there are 1,000 genes or 3 percent of the human genome that is dedicated to the nerve receptors that helps us to distinguish greater than 10,000 different smells. If any of those genes are defective, then you may not be able to distinguish certain smells. In fact, some people are born without the ability to distinguish smells at all. Not being able to smell at all is referred to anosmia. This is important not only because our sense of smell can enhance our moods and memories, but also because it can be a protective mechanism, as well. For example, we automatically tend to shy away from things that smell offensive to us as we may associate it with potential danger. Imagine not being able to smell a gas leak or detect the smell of smoke that can warn you of danger.

Even though we are told, time and time again, how inefficient the human sense of smell is, especially when compared to our cousins in the animal kingdom, one study conducted at the

University of California at Berkley demonstrated that human volunteers were able to track a scent up to thirty-three feet. Even more impressive is the fact that participants were able to improve this performance with practice.

Other potential causes of anosmia are growths in the nasal passages, such polyps, damage to the nerve receptors caused by chemicals or toxic substances such as pesticides, head trauma, neurological degenerative diseases, such as Alzheimer's and multiple sclerosis, old age, use of certain medications, such as certain antibiotics and antidepressants, and smoking.

Allergies: when good molecules go bad

Nasal allergies, referred to medically as allergic rhinitis, occurs in an estimated 10-30 percent of adults and 50 percent of children. It is anticipated that these individuals will experience at least four months per year of symptoms such as runny nose and nasal congestion. Those same molecules that can bring you the heavenly scent of a rose can also turn the rose into a potential nightmare if your nose has been primed to respond to these molecules as "not friendly." Molecules deemed by the nose as unfriendly will create a response designed to prevent these substances from entering any further into body. These molecules will activate immune cells in the nose and cause them to release inflammatory substances, such as histamines and leukotrienes, which cause tissues structures in nose to swell, leading to congestion and excessive mucous production. You may also find yourself sneezing incessantly. This is an example of a protective mechanism that can become over-responsive to substances that oftentimes mean "no harm."

What to do?

There are several steps that one can take to help reduce symptoms of allergic rhinitis. One approach is to inhibit the release of some of the substances that are released when immune cells are stimulated. Antihistamines, such as Benadryl and Zyrtec, work to prevent the release of histamines, and Singular works to inhibit the release of leukotrienes. By preventing the release of these inflammatory substances, many of the allergy symptoms, such as runny nose or nasal congestion, can be improved.

Other things that you can also try to remove some of allergens are the Nettie pot rinse with normal saline or just simply a normal saline rinse that can be easily found over the counter at your local drug store. Studies suggest that some substances like quercetin, found in onions, bromelain, found in pineapples, and omega-3's, found in flaxseed and fish may have anti-inflammatory properties that can help improve rhinitis symptoms. Certain vitamins such as vitamin C, vitamin B5, and vitamin B6 have also been shown in studies to support a healthy immune response, thus helping to keep the balance between too much and too little inflammation.

Short term inflammation is needed to heal, repair, and protect, but inappropriate or prolonged inflammation can be detrimental to the body and the nose. If you are experiencing persistent symptoms, you may need to visit an allergist to help determine if there are any triggers that can be avoided. If appropriate, your allergist may discuss with you allergy shots to help your immune system develop a tolerance to the identified allergens.

Other simple steps to consider are: removing clothing and shoes that may have accumulated allergens when you were outdoors, filtering the air that enters your home or keep a filtering device in your bedroom, covering the mattress and pillows with allergen resistant covers, and limiting the amount of carpet covered surfaces in your home.

Frequent Infections:

If you find yourself suffering from frequent sinus infections, you may be suffering from chronic allergies, chronic sinusitis, excessive stress, or an immune system that is hypo-functioning.

Your first step is to take a look at your lifestyle choices and nutritional habits. If you smoke or are exposed to second-hand smoke, take steps to stop and reduce exposure immediately. If your diet is void of healthy anti-oxidants or immune boosting foods such as spinach, winter squash, carrots, oranges, pumpkin seeds, healthy proteins such as salmon, turkey and beans, or healthy fats that help fight inflammation such as, avocadoes, sardines, and nuts, then take steps to adjust your diet. Eating this way may also help reduce the severity of your allergy symptoms, as well. Certain spices, such as turmeric and rosemary, are thought to have anti-inflammatory properties, as well.

Chronic infections may also represent anatomic anomalies such as septal deviation, a hard to eradicate organism such as a sinus infection caused by a fungus, or undertreated allergies. It is important for you to visit your physician to determine the underlying cause so that you can be treated appropriately.

Nutrient deficiency and sense of smell

Certain vitamin deficiencies, such as vitamin B12 deficiency, can cause neuropathy or damage to nerve cells including those in charge of smell, thus causing a decreased sense of smell. Not enough anti-oxidants in the diet, such as vitamin E, can leave nerve cells unprotected and susceptible to damage, thus once again, contributing to an impaired sense of smell. Several studies suggest that vitamin D has a positive impact on the immune system and can reduce the risk of contracting an upper respiratory infection.

Visit your Physician

If your symptoms persist, visit your physician as there might be other medical conditions that can cause loss of the sense of smell and/or persistent nasal congestion. If you are on medications that you suspect could be interfering with your sense of smell, discuss this with your physician, as well. At times, it may be necessary to see an Ear Nose and Throat specialist to rule out growths in your nasal cavity or sinuses. Also remember, certain neurological conditions such as Alzheimer's, Parkinson's and multiple sclerosis may have loss of the sense of smell as one of the first noticeable presenting symptom. You and your physician would need to work together to determine if your symptoms are caused by an underlying condition.

What about Pheromones?

What about the holy grail of attraction—pheromones? Do they exist, and if so, is human behavior influenced by them? Well, the jury is still out on this phenomenon. Yes, pheromones exist and play a significant role in the animal kingdom, and no, science is not definitive about whether humans are influenced by pheromones. Research, however, hints at some intriguing possibilities. One particular study, that I find very interesting, was performed by Claus Wedekind at the University of Bern in Switzerland. This study suggests that women may choose their mate based on genetic compatibility.

The study was based on research that showed that female mice chose mates that were genetically dissimilar to them. They were able to detect this difference by sniffing the urine of the male mice. The genetic material looked at was the MHC (**major histocompatibility complex),** the part of the gene that acts as the surveillance team to detect disease in the organism. With the MHC system, if Mom's MHC can detect disease B and Dad's MHC can detect disease A, then if offspring inherited one of each, his system would be able to detect disease A and B, thus allowing the immune system to get busy fighting off these diseases. This is certainly a leg up on the survival of the fittest scale. Another advantage of avoiding someone genetically similar is decreasing the risk of passing on a double dose of defective genes.

Of course, based on mouse research, one could understand how this would beg the question—does this happen in humans. A research study conducted at the University of Bern attempted to answer this question. In this research project one hundred college students were selected, males and females. The males were given strict instructions to avoid fragrances and spicy foods (anything that would interfere with their particular apocrine secretion) and were then given clean T-shirts to sleep in for two consecutive nights. The women were then given these T-shirts to sniff during their ovulation period as the female sense of smell is a little more acute during this time. They were asked to rate the shirts for "sexiness." Interestingly, the women rated sexiest the shirt of the male counterparts that had genetics that were different than their own. The shirts from the males with a higher degree of similarity to theirs were rated as much less appealing. Of course, this does not definitively answer the question, but it certainly makes one begin to appreciate the power of the nose.

Appreciating the Power of Your Nose:

When you look in the mirror, no matter the size, shape, or contour of your nose, I want you to recognize and appreciate the inherent power and sensuality of your nose. The size and the shape simply reflect the proud culture and nationality of those who came before you. It may be telling of their journey through harsh environments that required them to have more open or less open nasal passages. It may also be telling the story of the people they encountered along the way. Ultimately, it is the story of you, and you are more than enough right now. If you want to change something about your nose, don't wait to change it to feel good about yourself; feel good about yourself now. In the meantime, whether you contour, bejewel, or highlight your nose, know that your nose enhances your experience, and it does not define who you are.

My Personal Routine:

I learned to appreciate my nose a very long time ago. I have had it contoured and highlighted when I play dress up, and I appreciate the artistic difference it can make in photographs. However, what I appreciate the most about my nose is its ability to change the way I feel by simply inhaling a particular scent. I am a big fan of essential oils and use them frequently to lift my spirits, energize my brain, or relax into a sense of well-being. I can do all of this because of my ability to smell. For example, studies show that lavender and orange essential oils improve moods and decrease anxiety, and I have found that to be the case for me.

Keeping my nasal passages healthy and my sense of smell primed requires that I pay close attention to what I eat. I know that if I skimp on nutrients and antioxidants by eating primarily pita chips (my all-time favorite) and tortilla chips and salsa, I am going to start feeling run down, tired, and drained, and shortly thereafter, here comes a cold virus ready to set up shop in my nose. I know that if I start eating too many dairy products, then at some point, I start experiencing a little more nasal congestion.

If I feel myself getting rundown or tired, I immediately start paying attention to my diet and eating habits. I increase my vegetables and fruits such as spinach, oranges, carrots, and pumpkins to pump up my vitamin C, folic acid, and vitamin A. I eat apples, garlic, and onions for their high quercetin content and immune supporting ability. I start hydrating and avoiding the foods that I noticed in the past makes me feel not so well. I may take additional vitamin C and quercetin for a little more antihistamine support. If I am experiencing a little nasal congestion and/or dryness, I reach for the saline nasal irrigation solution to help relieve some of this symptomology. I may even reach for the old standby, the aroma of eucalyptus found in Vick's formula or lozenges as that may help to open my nasal passages.

Finally, every day, I find time to consciously connect to my breath. I sit or stand, take deep, long breaths, tuning in to the sensation of life and energy entering in through my nose, simultaneously soothing and energizing each cell of my body. I breathe in peace, joy, love, and I fully exhale life, passion, and creation. This regimen has been able to get me over the hump the majority of the time.

Sexercise:

Perhaps here is where you can remind yourself about the things you appreciate about your nose:

I love the scent of:

_____

_____Because it makes me feel

_____

I love the scent of:

_____

—

Because it reminds me of:

_____

Today, I chose to inhale: Check all that apply or do one a day. Feel free to add your own

- Peace
- Love
- Joy
- Gratitude
- My dreams

Chapter -7: Sexy Mouth

Healthy lips and beyond

The human race has only one really effective weapon, and that is laughter. ~ Mark Twain

If your mouth could talk—what would it say? Oh wait, vocal sounds and speech are emitted from the mouth, so your mouth can talk. But, are we missing the hidden messages our mouth might be whispering to us? When you dream of a sexy mouth, is the vision that jumps to your mind a sexy pout, full lips, lips shaped like a perfect bow, or some other vision that focuses on the size and the shape of your lips? Did you know that apart from your nails and eyes, your lips and tongue might be one of the best areas to check for telltale signs of nutrient deficiencies? For example, lack of Vitamin B2, known as riboflavin, can present as severely cracked lips. A vitamin B3 (niacin) deficiency can also present as cracked lips and a red, swollen tongue. Vitamin C deficiency can lead to swollen, fragile gums, and a pale tongue may be indicative of anemia from an iron deficiency.

As you can see, the mouth can reflect the health of your body. But, can the mouth be directly responsible for affecting the health of the body? Even though there is some controversy surrounding this issue, many studies are pointing to the fact that this is indeed the case. What, then, is the scoop on what makes the mouth sexy? In my opinion, a healthy mouth is a sexy mouth. Ask your dentist!

Healthy Lips

As I alluded to in the previous section, diet can play a significant role in the health and condition of your lips. Chapped lips can be a sign of more than just dry weather conditions. It can represent inadequacy of certain nutrients in the diet such as folic acid, essential fatty acids, vitamin B2, Vitamin B3, vitamin B12, biotin, and even vitamin C. The lack of these key nutrients can present as chapped lips, cracks or fissures at the corner of the mouth, and even a burning sensation of the lips and tongue, to name a few signs. This does not mean that you have to run out and take huge dosages of these vitamins. In fact, prior to adding supplements to your regimen, I recommend you speak with your physician as some supplements can interfere with medications and, in some cases, contribute to significant side effects and possible toxicities if taken in excess.

A healthy diet, however, can go a long way in creating a healthy mouth. A diet that has a mixture of eggs and yogurt, lean meats such as poultry and fish, colorful and green leafy vegetables such as carrots, broccoli, and spinach, fruits such as strawberries, bananas, and blueberries, nuts and seeds such as walnuts and pumpkin seeds, and whole grain products such as wheat germ can go a long way to keep those lips satiny smooth. If you are experiencing ongoing issues with dryness, sores or fissures to the lips, see your physician as other illnesses such as Chron's, eczema, and even skin cancers may have lip manifestations.

What about if your lips are healthy, and you just want them to be soft and more touchable? While I am not an aesthetician, most beauty experts agree on a few key points:

- Avoid licking lips constantly
- Use a lip balm or cream with SPF of at least 15 to protect lips from the damaging effects of UV rays from the sun
- Gentle exfoliation at night with a wash cloth may help to keep lips smooth and remove dead skin cells and makeup from the day
- Play close attention to the lipstick you apply on the lips as some can have very drying ingredients. There are even some concerns about heavy metal content in some lipsticks. Researchers at the University of California-Berkeley's School of Public Health expressed concerns about users that reapply lipstick frequently throughout the day as this may potentially increase exposure to small amounts of heavy metals they found in some products.

Healthy, Enticing Mouth- *A Journey beyond the Lips*

It would be difficult to find anyone who disagrees that a smile can literally transform the face. It is one of the magical tools that we have that can say welcome, I like you, be at ease, relax, and

I am happy to be where I am. Yes, an engaging smile can invite the world in, but a healthy mouth and fresh breath compels them to stick around a while and listen to what you have to say. So how do we accomplish this?

If we travel past the lips, we encounter our pearly whites, the teeth. As an adult, we have anywhere from twenty-eight to thirty-two teeth. Some are meant for biting and others for chewing. Our teeth, oftentimes, can determine how others judge us but, more importantly, how we judge ourselves. If we feel uncomfortable about the health or condition of our teeth, this frequently keeps us from expressing who we truly are and living and laughing out loud. We may hide behind our hands, bow our heads, or simply remain silent. In other words, we hold back a significant part of who we are, and the world is denied your sparkle and shine. Like it or not, a healthy mouth not only speaks volumes about our body, it also allow us to stand in the essence of who we are and speak our truth with confidence, thus enticing others to get a glimpse of the world the way we see it.

There was a girl I knew when I was about eleven years old. The thing that I recall most about her was the fact that whenever she laughed or spoke her hands immediately went up to her mouth and covered her lips, and she always looked down. As an eleven year old, I thought that was curious and came to the conclusion that she must be extremely shy. After all, that was something to which I could relate. This was until one day, in a rare moment, caught up in a moment of uncontrolled laughter, she did not place her hands over her lips, and I caught a glimpse of her front incisors. They were decayed beyond anything I had witnessed before and perhaps even after. I remember this today because this is perhaps one of the earliest realizations I had that our smile and our ability to laugh out loud can shape our personality and even our sense of who we are.

Taking Care of your Teeth and Gums—*Lead players in your smile*

The American Dental Association recommends brushing your teeth twice a day and flossing once a day to help prevent dental decay and disease. It is also recommended that you also change your toothbrush every three to four months as a frayed, mangled toothbrush won't clean teeth optimally and can potentially damage the gums. You should change your toothbrush after a bout with an upper respiratory infection.

Another component of good dental hygiene is flossing. Flossing helps remove food and plaque from between teeth, a place not accessible to the toothbrush. Plaque is formed by the action of bacteria in the mouth on the food that we eat. Plaque that is not removed then hardens and forms tartar. This buildup of plaque and tartar can then cause gum disease that can then lead to damage to the gums and bones, thus contributing to the premature loss of teeth. This inflammatory process is referred to as periodontal disease.

What is Periodontal Disease?

Periodontal disease refers to conditions that impact the health of the gums or gingiva, the connective tissue that holds the teeth into the socket and bone or alveolar that anchors the teeth. Therefore, severe periodontal disease can lead to premature loss of teeth in adults. In fact, it is the leading cause of tooth loss in adults. Some studies suggest that periodontal disease may even contribute to or exacerbate systemic conditions such as heart disease.

The first stage of gum disease is the inflammation of the gums. This is referred to as gingivitis. This stage, according to the ADA, is reversible. If it is not treated, then it can progress to periodontal disease that is not reversible. Periodontal means that the inflammation has spread from the gums to the bone and the tissue that connects the teeth to the bone. This inflammation can destroy these structures leading to tooth loss.

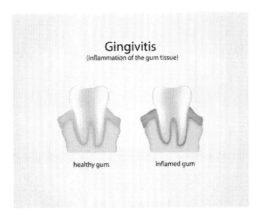

Gingivitis
(inflammation of the gum tissue)

healthy gum   inflamed gum

Signs and Symptoms of Periodontal Disease:

So how would you know if you have signs and symptoms of early or later periodontal disease? Some early signs of inflammation are redness and tenderness of the gums, gums that bleed easily, gums pulling away from the teeth, bad breath or bad taste in the mouth, and teeth that are lose or shaking. Any of these signs and/or symptoms should prompt an immediate appointment with your dentist. Of course, regular visits to the dentist can help identify these issues before they become irreversible.

What Causes Periodontitis?

It is thought that periodontitis starts with the accumulation of plaque. If we recall, plaque is formed when the sugar and starches in the foods that you eat interact with the bacteria in your mouth. This reaction forms a sticky film that deposits and builds up along the gum line. Plaque can be removed by brushing and flossing, but if left to accumulate on the teeth for days, it can interact with the minerals in your saliva and harden to a substance called tartar. Tartar is not so easily removed by brushing and flossing and usually has to be removed by the dentist with lots of scraping. I am sure many of us can attest to the sometimes uncomfortable nature of this process. If tartar is allowed to build up between the teeth and the gum line, it becomes a magnate for more bacteria, thus perpetuating the process. This build of plaque, tartar, and bacteria starts generating a lot of inflammation. At first, you may just notice redness and irritation of the gums (gingivitis), but as tartar builds up and the inflammation and infection progresses, deeper pockets start forming between the teeth and the gums, allowing the inflammation to impact the deeper periodontal structures. This can then lead to destruction of bony tissue and connective tissue that anchors the teeth leading to tooth loss.

Electric vs. Manual:

We are now aware that we should brush twice and floss once daily for optimum teeth and gum protection, but with so many choices of toothbrushes and forms of floss, it begs the question— which is best? First, the ADA formal position is it does not matter if one uses a manual toothbrush or an electric toothbrush. They recommend using a soft toothbrush and focus more on brushing techniques. In my opinion, sound advice.

However, let's explore the data on electric versus manual. A review published in the *Journal of Dentistry* in March 2004 reviewed studies that compared manual toothbrushes to powered or electric toothbrushes. They measured effectiveness by the amount of plaque buildup and on the health of the gums or the amount of gingivitis. They found that manual and most forms of powered brushes performed very similarly. One form of the electric toothbrush, the rotary, oscillatory toothbrush, was found to be slightly superior in reducing plaque and gingivitis. In the long run (greater than three months) this form reduced gingivitis by as much as 17 percent.

What about the ultrasonic toothbrush, is that superior to the oscillation, rotation brush? The *American Journal of Dentistry* published a review in April of 2013 that looked at studies that compared manual versus ultrasound versus oscillation, rotation toothbrushes. The verdict—the oscillation, rotation toothbrush still maintained its superiority when it came to plaque removal on those hard to reach areas. The take home point, though, was all brushes were effective for plaque removal. So, whichever one you choose, just brush twice a day for the recommended two minutes for a healthy smile.

Most of us, hopefully, can commit to flossing once a day, but can we decide which floss is best for us? Should we stick with the old standby or graduate up to the new electric water picks? Well, here is some important information that may help you decide what is best for you. The first piece of information is that the ADA recommends flossing daily. Now, while some studies suggest that using a water pic may be superior to strand flossing in preventing gingivitis, there might be advantages to both. Strand floss may be better at removing plaque in between teeth while water pics maybe more beneficial for those with sensitive gums and definitely those with braces as a strand would be difficult to maneuver. The ADA recommends when using manual floss the most effect technique is to curve it against the shape of the teeth at the gum line. For a better visual, visit http://www.mouthhealthy.org/en/az-topics/f/flossing. This is also a discussion you would want to have with your dentist as he can help you to determine which technique and modality would be more suited to your individual needs.

What about the effectiveness of antiseptic mouth rinse? After all, every other commercial on the television or the radio challenges us to banish bad breath forever or at least twenty-four hours by enjoyably and playfully swishing around a tasty mouth wash for a few minutes. Is this truth or fiction? Well, according to the *Journal of Dental Hygiene* February 2013, some mouth washes can be effective at controlling plaque and gingivitis. The most effective ingredients were essential oils eucalyptol, thymol and menthol, and 0.12 percent chlorhexidine gluconate. Mouthwashes containing cetylpyridinium chloride did not seem to be as effective. Now, the jury is still out on whether this translates into reduced occurrence of periodontal disease, but sometimes, it just feels great to have that fresh breath feeling.

Super Nutrients that prevent Gingivitis: *Out of the box thinking, beyond mouthwash and toothpaste*

Now, let me start by saying that no amount of supplements will take the place of good dental hygiene as mentioned above. Just like a multivitamin cannot take the place of healthy diet, nothing mentioned below can take the place of brushing, flossing, and regular visits to your dentist. Now, let us take a look at studies suggesting several substances that may be helpful adjuncts to help keep your gums in great shape.

Several studies published in the *Journal of Periodontology* in the 1980's suggest that folic acid as a mouth rinse may help to reduce the occurrence of gingivitis. It is important to note that the taking folic acid orally or in pill form did not seem to create the same improvement.

Another vitamin that seems to have an impact on oral health is vitamin D. Individuals with low Vitamin D levels had higher incidence of gingivitis as noted by Dietrich, et al. in the *Journal of Clinical Nutrition* in September 2005. While this does not prove causation, it might be just another reason to be sure that your vitamin D level is adequate. Also, a review of twenty-four clinical trials looking at the effect of vitamin D on the health of the teeth published in December issue of the *Journal of Nutrition Reviews* came to the conclusion that vitamin D decreased the risk of developing cavities. This is yet another reason to love sunshine.

What about herbal remedies? We already noted that essential oils such as thymol (derived from thyme), found in Listerine, have been shown to decrease gingivitis. In 2002, a study utilizing pycnogenol gum found that it significantly reduced plaque buildup and symptoms of gingivitis such as bleeding gums. Xylitol, a sugar found naturally in some fruits, such as strawberries, takes it a step further; it actually reduces the bacteria that causes plaque and forms the acid that can erode the tooth and lead to cavities. Xylitol can be found in toothpaste, as well as chewing gum. In fact, one study looking at toothpaste that contained fluoride alone versus toothpaste that contained both fluoride and xylitol, found that over a three year period the children using the xylitol toothpaste developed less cavities than those who used fluoride toothpaste.

If the bacteria in the mouth cause cavities, what if we attempt to replace the cavity causing bacteria in the mouth with a friendlier strain of bacteria that does not cause cavities? Several studies using several strains of probiotics (yes, these guys to the rescue again) have shown that just this, indeed, may be possible. Some of probiotics studied were L. Reuteri, S. Salivarius, and Bacillus coagulans. They all seem to compete extremely well with one of the bad boys of cavities, *Streptococcus mutans,* kicking it off the tooth enamel so it can do no harm. I know it all seems like some science fiction war, but in this war, there are some bacteria on our side.

Another titan in the war against the cavity causing Streptococcus mutans is green tea extract. In fact, the extracts from green tea, epigallocatechin gallate (EGCg) and epicatechin gallate (ECg), have been shown to suppress this bacterium by decreasing its ability to feed on sugar, thus neutralizing its ability to form plaque. Score another one for Mother Nature.

Process of Cavity Formation:

When bacteria consume the sugar from the foods we eat, they form plaque and then begin to secrete an acid. This acid, if allowed to be in contact with the tooth for an extended period of time, will begin to erode the enamel or hard outer structure of the tooth. This creates a hole in the tooth that allows bacteria to enter and continue the process. Bacteria like Streptococcus mutans use the enzyme glucosyl transferase to feed on sugar, thus creating acid as a byproduct. Beware that sugars refers to carbohydrates, especially simple carbohydrates found in foods such as rice, potatoes, and pasta. Green tea extract works to decrease the activity of this enzyme, thus decreasing these bacteria's ability to cause cavities.

It is thought that acidic foods can also start this process of enamel erosion leading to cavities. The good news is that a healthy flow of saliva can begin the process of washing away the acid from the surface of the tooth. Individuals who suffer from dry mouth syndrome lose this benefit of saliva and so are more predisposed to the occurrence of cavities.

It is recommended by most dentists that you visit the dentist at least twice a year for regular dental cleaning and monitoring of the health of your teeth and gums. Also, at those times, you are likely to get fluoride treatment to enhance the strength of the enamel of your teeth. Protecting your enamel is one of the key ways to protect the integrity and longevity of your teeth.

What about the tongue?

The tongue is an organ made up primarily of muscle. Yes, the tongue is basically a muscle that can taste. Amazing! The bumps you see on your tongue are called papillae. Surrounding these papillae are taste buds that are primarily nerve bundles that connect to the brain. We have all heard about or seen the taste maps that tell us that certain areas of the tongue are responsible for detecting a particular taste such as bitter, sour, sweet, and salty. The truth is all parts of the tongue are capable of detecting all the different taste. Most importantly, without the tongue, we would not be able to swallow, chew, or speak!

Did you know that the tongue is also used in many cultures to determine the health of the body? In fact, this is one of the major diagnostic tools in Traditional Chinese Medicine (TCM). While it is not considered a major diagnostic tool in western or allopathic medicine, we can still suspect some deficiencies and diagnosis based on examination of the tongue. For example, a smooth tongue may be indicative of vitamin B12 deficiency, a pale tongue may point to anemia, and a reddish inflamed tongue may point to niacin, vitamin B12, or folic acid deficiency. A tremulous or uncontrollable tongue may reflect trouble in the nervous system, anxiety, or maybe even an overactive thyroid. As you can begin to appreciate, the tongue is an extremely important structure in the mouth that deserves just as much attention and care as the teeth. So, when your physician examines your tongue, remember, she may glean some important information about the health of your body.

How important is brushing or scraping the tongue in maintaining good oral hygiene? Well, according to researchers, cleaning the tongue is an important part of maintaining fresh breath, at least temporarily. Keep in mind there may also be other causes of bad breath, so if bad breath persists, see your doctor.

Lifestyle Habits to Promote Healthy Teeth, Gums and Tongue:

As already mentioned earlier, diet is an important part of a healthy mouth, but were you aware that habits such as smoking can have a negative impact on the health of your mouth? This damage is not limited to bad breath and discolored teeth. Research in the field has linked smoking with the increased occurrence of gingivitis, periodontal disease, and loss of teeth. In fact, a study published in the *Journal of Periodontal* May 2000, goes as far as to say it may be responsible for half of the cases of periodontal disease in the United States today. Not only do smokers have a much higher incidence of periodontal disease, they also seem to respond less favorably to treatment. This is certainly a double whammy. The good news is that smoking cessation seems to reduce the risk of periodontal disease.

What about stress? Stress seems to have impact on everything else, but does it also impact the health of our mouth? It seems the answer to this question is—YES, stress seems to increase the risk of gum disease! Several theories abound. One theory is that stress may lead us to develop and/or perpetuate harmful habits in an attempt to cope. Habits such as smoking, turning to sugary foods, excessive alcohol use, and perhaps even just neglecting proper dental hygiene can escalate the development of gingivitis and periodontal disease. Another potential culprit is the excess cortisol produced by chronic stress. Persistently elevated cortisol levels can lead to immunity suppression and a tendency to weaken bone tissue.

The Mouth and Your General Health:

Can poor dental hygiene contribute or exacerbate diseased states? Several recent studies are pointing strongly in that direction. We should not be surprised by this; after all, individuals with significant valve disorders or replacements have always been treated with antibiotics prior to dental procedures due to concerns that bacteria from the mouth may infect the heart valves. Studies are suggesting that those same bacteria may also contribute toward causing a blockage in the arteries that supply the oxygen to the heart. This blockage can then potentially lead to a heart attack.

An article published in the *National Institute of Dental and Craniofacial Research* (NIDCR) gives us insight as to how this can occur. These researchers found that a bacterium in the mouth called Porphyromonas gingivalis was able to activate specific immune cells (monocytes) and cause them to stick to the clotting protein called fibrinogen. This clotting protein then attached itself to the lining of blood vessels. Since fibrinogen facilitates the formation of clots, this can potentially lead to blockage of blood flow to heart, thus leading to a heart attack. In another study published in the *Journal of Circulation*, researchers also found that individuals with a higher percentage of four particular strains of bacteria that caused periodontal disease also had an increase in the walls of their carotid arteries, one of the main set of vessels that supply blood and oxygen to the brain. While association does not equal causation, these results would certainly seem to be consistent with the clotting protein theory. I am sure that further studies will help us shed more light on this matter. However, the thought that what goes on in one part of the body having an impact on the other parts of the body should not surprise us.

Your Healthy Mouth Routine:

It is important that you develop a routine that works for you. The basics are brushing teeth twice a day with soft bristles to protect the enamel and flossing at least once a day. In my opinion, the type of brush you choose and method of flossing you choose is a personal choice. They are all effective when used as recommended. You may also choose to add an antiseptic mouthwash to your routine after discussion with your dentist.

Example routine:

After experimenting with toothbrushes, floss, and mouthwashes, devise a routine that keeps your mouth and your dentist happy. As always, I encourage you to have an honest conversation with your dental specialist about your habits and health so you can determine the best routine for you.

Start with brushing your teeth and tongue the recommended twice daily and floss nightly. Experiment with manual versus rotary, oscillatory toothbrushes to see which one keeps your mouth fresher longer and make flossing a little easier. If you choose a water floss, consider adding a capful of your favorite mouthwash to the water. Then, follow with manual flossing to keep plaque formation to a minimum. Consider augmenting your dental routine with several sprays of xylitol daily or a probiotic lozenge containing specific strains used in dental studies. Keep tabs on how you are doing by following up with your dentist every six months. This is an example of a basic routine that could reduce malodorous breath, keep plaque formation to a minimum, prevent cavities, and keep your quirky smile healthy and appealing.

Sexercise:

A sexy back activity

You deserve to laugh out loud, turn the world on with your smile, and have a healthy and happy mouth. If you feel that aesthetically you do not have a smile that you are willing or excited to share, then change it without judgement from yourself or others. There are many truly gifted dentists, orthodontists, and dental surgeons who are willing and able to do so. On the other hand, if you love the slight gap between your teeth or simply adore that one quirky crooked incisor, then embrace that, and show the world the uniqueness that is you. Go ahead, radiate your confidence with that amazing smile and that infectious laugh. Highlight those lips with the most amazing pop of red because you will no longer shy away from speaking your truth!

The one thing I love about my smile is:

_____

_____

_____

The one thing I can do to improve or enhance my smile or my oral hygiene is:

_____

_____

_____

Today, I will speak my truth about:

_____

_____

_____

_____

The information provided within this book is for general informational purposes only. While we try to keep the information up-to-date and correct, there are no representations or warranties, express or implied, about the completeness, accuracy, reliability, suitability or availability with respect to the information, products, services, or related graphics contained in this book for any purpose. Any use of this information is at your own risk.

Neither the author nor the publisher is responsible for actions based on the content of this book. It is not the purpose of this book to include all information about a healthy wellness program. This book is not intended as a substitute for the medical advice of physicians. The reader should regularly consult a physician in matters relating to his/her health and particularly with respect to any symptoms that may require diagnosis or medical attention.

In addition, information and research are continuously changing so please understand what is printed here may not be the most current information available.

If you light a lamp for somebody it will also brighten your path ~

Buddha

My passion has always been to inform and educate because I do believe in the power of knowledge. I realize that I cannot provide all the answers to the questions you may have but, if I can, in some small way, help you to ignite the spark that each of us has within then, the hours spent putting information to paper was worth it.

You may have noticed that this book is titled volume 1. I decided to create a two part series instead of putting all the information into one large book because I did not want to induce memories of the large novels you had to read in high school or college. My goal was to create a user friendly series that was easy to navigate yet informative. So in the next part of the series, I will discuss why being heart healthy is absolutely necessary for that healthy glow, how to get off the hormonal roller coaster train so that your over fifty is fabulous and how to minimize inflammation to help you to lose weight.

Healthy and Sexy References

BRAIN/MENTAL

Jin TaeHong et. al. Neuroprotective effect of green tea extract in experimental ischemia-reperfusion brain injury: Brain Research Bulletin Volume 53, Issue 6, December 2000, Pages 743-749

Sun-Edelstein, Christina MD Clinical Foods and Supplements in the Management of Migraine Headaches, Journal of Pain: June 2009 - Volume 25 - Issue 5 - pp 446-452

Paola Schiapparelli Non-pharmacological approach to migraine prophylaxis: part II, Neurological Sciences June 2010, Volume 31, Issue 1 Supplement, pp 137-139

P. S. Sándor Efficacy of coenzyme Q10 in migraine prophylaxis: A randomized controlled trial Neurology February 22, 2005 vol. 64 no. 4 713-715

Andrew D. Hershey MD, Coenzyme Q10 Deficiency and Response to Supplementation in Pediatric and Adolescent Migraine Headache: The Journal of Head and Face Pain, Volume 47, Issue 1, pages 73–80, January 2007

R. B. Lipton, MD Petasites hybridus root (butterbur) is an effective preventive treatment for migraine Neurology December 28, 2004 vol. 63 no. 12 2240-2244

Sirichai Chayasirisobhon MD, et. al. Use of a Pine Bark Extract and Antioxidant Vitamin Combination Product as Therapy for Migraine in Patients Refractory to Pharmacologic Medication Headache: The Journal of Head and Face Pain, Volume 46, Issue 5, pages 788–793, May 2006

Michael Berka, Neurostimulatory and Neuroablative Treatments for Depression: Biological Psychiatry Volume 64, Issue 6, 15 September 2008, Pages 468–475

Rendeiro C, Dietary levels of pure flavonoids improve spatial memory performance and increase hippocampal brain-derived neurotrophic factor: <u>PLoS One.</u> 2013 May 28;8(5):e63535.

Janice K. Kiecolt-Glasera Brain, Omega-3 supplementation lowers inflammation and anxiety in medical students: A randomized controlled trial: Behavior, and Immunity Volume 25, Issue 8, November 2011, Pages 1725–1734

Lee ST1 Panax ginseng enhances cognitive performance in Alzheimer disease Alzheimer Dis Assoc Disord. 2008 Jul-Sep;22(3):222-6..

Maesako M1, Uemura K, Continuation of exercise is necessary to inhibit high fat diet-induced β-amyloid deposition and memory deficit in amyloid precursor protein transgenic mice: PLoS One. 2013 Sep 4;8(9):e72796.

Morris, MC1 Dietary fats and the risk of incident Alzheimer

disease. Arch Neurol. 2003 Feb;60(2):194-200.

K. Chandrasekhar, A Prospective, Randomized Double-Blind,

Placebo-Controlled Study of Safety and Efficacy of a High-

Concentration Full-Spectrum Extract of Ashwagandha Root in

Reducing Stress and Anxiety in Adults, Indian J Psychol Med. 2012

Jul;34(3):255-62

Janice K., Kiecolt-Glaser Close Relationships, Inflammation, and

Health: Neurosci Biobehav Rev. Sep 2010; 35(1): 33–38.

Weinstein G Serum brain-derived neurotrophic factor and the risk

for dementia: the Framingham Heart Study JAMA Neurol. 2014

Jan;71(1):55-61.

Nicolas Cherbuin, PhD, Higher normal fasting plasma glucose is

associated with hippocampal atrophy. The PATH Study

Neurology September 4, 2012 vol. 79 no. 10 1019-1026

Francis ST, The effect of flavanol-rich cocoa on the fMRI response to a cognitive task in healthy young people: J Cardiovasc Pharmacol. 2006;47 Suppl 2:S215-20.

Munafò MR, The serotonin transporter gene and depression Depress Anxiety. 2012 Nov;29(11):915-7.

Kaneko H, Proof of the mysterious efficacy of ginseng: basic and clinical trials: clinical effects of medical ginseng, Korean red ginseng: specifically, its anti-stress action for prevention of disease: J Pharmacol Sci. 2004;95:158–162

Huibo Shao, Hormone therapy and Alzheimer disease dementia: New findings from the Cache County Study WNL. Neurology, October 24, 2012 Henriette van Praag Trends Neurosci. 2009 May; 32(5): 283–290.

.

Effects of nicotine chewing gum on a real-life motor task: a kinematic analysis of handwriting movements in smokers and non-smokers. Psychopharmacology (Berl). 2004 Apr;173(1-2):49-56. Epub 2003 Dec 11

Newhouse P, Kellar K, et al. Nicotine treatment of mild cognitive impairment: A 6-month double-blind pilot clinical trial. Neurology 2012; 78:91-101.

Newhouse PA, Potter AS. Acute nicotine improves cognitive deficits in young adults with attention deficit/hyperactivity disorder. Pharmacol Biochem Behav 2008;88(4):407-417.

Quik, M, Nicotine reduces levadopa-induced dyskinesias in lesioned monkeys. Ann Neurol 2007;62(6):588-596

Tariq M, Khan HA, Elfaki I, et al. Neuroprotective effect of nicotine against 3-nitropropionic acid (3-NP)-induced experimental

Huntington's disease in rats. Brain Res Bull 2005 Sep 30;67(1-2):161-168.

Federation of American Societies for Experimental Biology. "Want a good night's sleep in the New Year? Quit smoking." ScienceDaily. ScienceDaily, 2 January 2014.

Stoschitzky K, Influence of beta-blockers on melatonin release. Eur J Clin Pharmacol. 1999 Apr;55(2):111-5.

Y. M. Kuo, Deprivation of pantothenic acid elicits a movement disorder and azoospermia in a mouse model of pantothenate kinase-associated neurodegeneration: Journal of Inherited Metabolic Disease June 2007, Volume 30, Issue 3, pp 310-317

Zhoura Lakroun, Oxidative stress and brain mitochondria swelling induced by endosulfan and protective role of quercetin in rat: Environmental Science and Pollution Research, February 2015

Dr. Lukas PezawasSource: Depression Gene May Weaken Mood-regulating Circuit NIH/National Institute Of Mental Health Date: 10 May 2005

Sandyk R1, Kay SR The relationship of pineal calcification and melatonin secretion to the pathophysiology of tardive dyskinesia and Tourette's syndrome Int J Neurosci. 1991 Jun;58(3-4):215-47.

Cardinali DP, Therapeutic application of melatonin in mild cognitive impairment Am J Neurodegener Dis. 2012;1(3):280-91.

Beuckmann CT, Orexins: from neuropeptides to energy homeostasis and sleep/wake regulation J Mol Med (Berl). 2002 Jun;80(6):329-42.

Ohno K, Sakurai T, Orexin neuronal circuitry: role in the regulation of sleep and wakefulness Front Neuroendocrinol. 2008 Jan;29(1):70-87.

Brian C. Trainor, Oxytocin receptors in the anteromedial bed nucleus of the stria terminalis promote stress-induced social avoidance in females. *Biological Psychiatry*, 2017

Turhan Canli, Sex differences in the neural basis of emotional memories Proceedings of the National Academy of Sciences of the United States of America vol. 99 no. 16

Seung-SchikYoo, The human emotional brain without sleep — a prefrontal amygdala disconnect Current biology Volume 17, Issue 20, 23 October 2007, Pages R877-R878

Jennifer S.Stevens, Sex differences in brain activation to emotional stimuli: A meta-analysis of neuroimaging studies: Neuropsychologia Volume 50, Issue 7, June 2012, Pages 1578-1593

Jeremy W. Gawryluk, Decreased levels of glutathione, the major brain antioxidant, in post-mortem prefrontal cortex from patients with psychiatric disorders: *International Journal of Neuropsychopharmacology*, Volume 14, Issue 1, 1 February 2011, Pages 123–130

P.V.Magalhães N-acetyl cysteine add-on treatment for bipolar II disorder: a subgroup analysis of a randomized placebo-controlled trial: Journal of Affective Disorders Volume 129, Issues 1–3, March 2011, Pages 317-320

L. Feng, Tea consumption reduces the incidence of neurocognitive disorders: Findings from the Singapore longitudinal aging study. The Journal of Nutrition, Health & Aging, 2016; 20 (10)

Kara J. Blacker, Dual N-back Versus Complex Span Working Memory Training. Journal of Cognitive Enhancement, 2017

Jackob N. Keynan, Limbic Activity Modulation Guided by Functional Magnetic Resonance Imaging–Inspired

Electroencephalography Improves Implicit Emotion

Regulation. Biological Psychiatry, 2016; 80 (6): 490

Annette Maczurek, Lipoic acid as an anti-inflammatory and

neuroprotective treatment for Alzheimer's disease, Advanced Drug

Delivery Reviews Volume 60, Issues 13–14, October–November

2008, Pages 1463-1470

Ramlackhansingh AF, Inflammation after trauma: microglial

activation and traumatic brain injury. Ann Neurol 2011, 70:374–

383.

Kavon Rezai-Zadeh, Green Tea Epigallocatechin-3-Gallate (EGCG)

Modulates Amyloid Precursor Protein Cleavage and Reduces

Cerebral Amyloidosis in Alzheimer Transgenic Mice Journal of

Neuroscience 21 September 2005, 25 (38) 8807-8814;

Theresa M. Harrison, Superior Memory and Higher Cortical

Volumes in Unusually Successful Cognitive Aging: Journal of the

International Neuropsychological Society, 2012

LiisaTyrväinen, The influence of urban green environments on

stress relief measures: A field experiment; Journal of Environmental

Psychology Volume 38, June 2014, Pages 1-9

Richard M.Ryan NettaWeinstein Vitalizing effects of being

outdoors and in nature Journal of Environmental Psychology

Volume 30, Issue 2, June 2010, Pages 159-168

Oppezzo, M., & Schwartz, D. L. (2014). Give your ideas some legs:

The positive effect of walking on creative thinking. *Journal of

Experimental Psychology: Learning, Memory, and Cognition,*

40(4), 1142-1152.

Plante, T. G., Cage, C., Clements, S., & Stover, A. (2006).

Psychological benefits of exercise paired with virtual reality:

Outdoor exercise energizes whereas indoor virtual exercise relaxes. International Journal of Stress Management, *13*(1), 108-117.

Kara J. Blacker, Serban Negoita, Joshua B. Ewen, Susan M. Courtney. N-back Versus Complex Span Working Memory Training. Journal of Cognitive Enhancement, 2017;

Jackob N. Keynan, Yehudit Meir-Hasson; Limbic Activity Modulation Guided by Functional Magnetic Resonance Imaging–Inspired Electroencephalography Improves Implicit Emotion Regulation. Biological Psychiatry, 2016; 80 (6)

HAIR:

Isabelle C. Hay, MRCP; Randomized Trial of AromatherapySuccessful Treatment for Alopecia Areata *Arch Dermatol. Nov* 1998;134(11):1349-1352

Ji Young Oh, Peppermint Oil Promotes Hair Growth without Toxic Signs: Toxicol Res. 2014 Dec; 30(4): 297–304.

J.van der Donk, Quality of life and maladjustment associated with hair loss in women with alopecia androgenetica: Social Science & Medicine Volume 38, Issue 1, January 1994, Pages 159-163

Lee BH, Hair Growth-Promoting Effects of Lavender Oil in C57BL/6 Mice: Toxicol Res. 2016 Apr;32(2):103-8.

Eva M.J. Peters Probing the Effects of Stress Mediators on the Human Hair Follicle Substance P Holds Central Position: Am J Pathol. 2007 Dec; 171(6): 1872–1886.

Syed Suhail, Amin Alopecia areata: A review Journal of the Saudi Society of Dermatology & Dermatologic Surgery Volume 17, Issue 2, July 2013, Pages 37–45

E Buhl, Minoxidil's action in hair follicles J Invest Dermatol, 96 (Suppl) (1991), pp. 73S–74S

M Ericson, K Binstock, A Guanche, et al. Differential expression of substance P in perifollicular scalp blood vessels and nerves after topical therapy with capsaicin 0.075% (Zostrix HP) in controls and patients with extensive alopecia areata, J Invest Dermatol, 112 (1999), p. 65

N. Barahmani1Serum T helper 1 cytokine levels are greater in patients with alopecia areata regardless of severity or atopyIssue Clinical and Experimental Dermatology Volume 35, Issue 4, pages 409–416, June 2010

Nancy Todes-Taylor, M.D T cell subpopulaions in alopecia areata Journal of the American Academy of Dermatology Volume 11, Issue 2, Part 1, August 1984, Pages 216–223

Aditya K Gupta, MD, FRCPCa Oral cyclosporine for the treatment of alopecia areata : A clinical and immunohistochemical analysis Journal of the American Academy of Dermatology Volume 22, Issue 2, Part 1, February 1990, Pages 242–250

Luis A. Garza Prostaglandin D2 Inhibits Hair Growth and Is Elevated in Bald Scalp of Men with Androgenetic Alopecia Science Translational Medicine Vol 4, Issue 126 21 March 2012

Satoshi Yamamoto, Stimulation of Hair Growth by Topical Application of FK506, a Potent Immunosuppressive Agent Hong Jiang Journal of Investigative Dermatology, Volume 102, Issue 2, February 1994, Pages 160–164

Davis MG A novel cosmetic approach to treat thinning hair: Br J Dermatol. 2011 Dec;165 Suppl 3:24-30.

Deloche C., Low iron stores: a risk factor for excessive hair loss in non-menopausal women: Eur J Dermatol. 2007 Nov-Dec;17(6):507-12. Epub 2007 Oct 19.

Moeinvaziri M, Iron status in diffuse telogen hair loss among women. Acta Dermatovenerol Croat. 2009;17(4):279-84.

Adiam W Bahta, Premature Senescence of Balding Dermal Papilla Cells In Vitro Is Associated with p16INK4a Expression: Journal of Investigative Dermatology (2008) 128, 1088–1094.

Mizushima Y, Topical application of superoxide dismutase cream. Drugs Exp Clin Res. 1991;17(2):127-31.

Rushton DH, Nutritional factors and hair loss, Clin Exp Dermatol. 2002 Jul;27(5):396-404.

The Effect of Methylsulfonylmethane on Hair Growth Promotion of Magnesium Ascorbyl Phosphate for the Treatment of Alopecia

Biomolecules & Therapeutics - BIOMOL THER 01/2009; 17(3):241-248.

Wickett RR1, Kossmann E Effect of oral intake of choline-stabilized orthosilicic acid on hair tensile strength and morphology in women with fine hair, Arch Dermatol Res. 2007 Dec;299(10):499-505.

Takahashi T, The first clinical trial of topical application of procyanidin B-2 to investigate its potential as a hair growing agent Phytother Res. 2001 Jun;15(4):331-6.

Trüeb RM, Association between smoking and hair loss: another opportunity for health education against smoking, Dermatology. 2003;206(3):189-91.

Zayed AA, Smokers' hair: Does smoking cause premature hair graying? Indian Dermatol Online J. 2013 Apr;4(2):90-2.

Fischer TW, Topical melatonin for treatment of androgenetic alopecia: Int J Trichology. 2012 Oct;4(4):236-45.

Senile hair graying: H_2O_2-mediated oxidative stress affects human hair color by blunting methionine sulfoxide repair FASEB J July 2009 23:2065-2075; published ahead of print February 23, 2009,

Fischer TW, Melatonin increases anagen hair rate in women with androgenetic alopecia or diffuse alopecia: results of a pilot randomized controlled trial: Br J Dermatol. 2004 Feb;150(2):341-5.

Oura H, Adenosine increases anagen hair growth and thick hairs in Japanese women with female pattern hair loss: a pilot, double-blind, randomized, placebo-controlled trial: J Dermatol. 2008 Dec;35(12):763-7.

Takahashi T, Investigation of the topical application of procyanidin oligomers from apples to identify their potential use as a hair-growing agent: J Cosmet Dermatol. 2005 Dec;4(4):245-9

Zappacosta AR, Reversal of baldness in patient receiving minoxidil for hypertension: *N Engl J Med* 1980; 303: 1480-1.

Uno H, Cappas A, Brigham P., Action of topical minoxidil in the bald stump-tailed macaque: *J Am Acad Dermatol* 1987; 16: 657-68.

Scheinfeld N., A review of hormonal therapy for female pattern (androgenic) alopecia: Dermatol Online J. 2008 Mar 15;14(3):1.

Camacho-Martínez FM, Hair loss in women Semin Cutan: Med Surg. 2009 Mar;28(1):19-32.

Arase S, Co-culture of human hair follicles and dermal papillae in a collagen matrix: J Dermatol. 1990 Nov;17(11):667-76.

Hwang TL, Magnesium ascorbyl phosphate and coenzyme Q10 protect keratinocytes against UVA irradiation by suppressing glutathione depletion: Mol Med Rep. 2012 Aug;6(2):375-8.

RL Glaser, Improvement in scalp hair growth in androgen-deficient women treated with testosterone: a questionnaire study, Br J Dermatol. Feb 2012; 166(2): 274–278

I. Ali, Physiological Changes in Scalp, Facial and Body Hair after the Menopause, The British Journal of Dermatology The British Journal of Dermatology. 2011;14(3):508-513

T.W. Fischer, Clinical and laboratory investigations: Differential effects of caffeine on hair shaft elongation, matrix and outer root sheath keratinocyte proliferation, and TGF-β2-/IGF-1-mediated regulation of hair cycle in male and female human hair follicles in vitro. British Journal of Dermatology

Department of Dermatology and Allergology, Friedrich-Schiller-University, Jena, Germany: Effect of caffeine and testosterone on the proliferation of human hair follicles in vitro. International Journal of Dermatology (Impact Factor: 1.34). 02/2007; 46(1):27-35.

Toshihiko Hibino, Role of TGF-beta2 in the human hair cycle Journal of Dermatological: Science Volume 35, Issue 1, June 2004, Pages 9-18

Kayampilly PP1 Endocrinology. Stimulatory effect of insulin on 5alpha-reductase type 1 (SRD5A1) expression through an Akt-dependent pathway in ovarian granulosa cells 2010 Oct;151(10):5030-7.

Dong Ha Kim, M.D., Successful Treatment of Alopecia Areata with Topical Calcipotriol: Ann Dermatol. 2012 Aug; 24(3): 341–344.

Çerman AA, Topical Calcipotriol Therapy for Mild-to-Moderate Alopecia Areata: A Retrospective Study J Drugs Dermatol. 2015 Jun;14(6):616-20.

PratimaKarnik, et. al. Hair Follicle Stem Cell-Specific *PPARγ* Deletion Causes Scarring Alopecia Journal of Investigative Dermatology Volume 129, Issue 5, May 2009, Pages 1243-1257

Gerulf Rieger, The Eyes Have It: Sex and Sexual Orientation Differences in Pupil Dilation Patterns PLOS ONE August 03, 2012

Cecilia I. Calero, Allosteric Modulation of Retinal GABA Receptors by Ascorbic Acid, The Journal of Neuroscience, 29 June 2011, 31(26): 9672-9682;

Kazuhiro Tokuda, MD, Effects of ascorbic acid on UV light-mediated photoreceptor damage in isolated rat retina Exp Eye Res. Mar 2007; 84(3): 537–543.

Babizhayev MA[1], Burke L N-Acetylcarnosine sustained drug delivery eye drops to control the signs of ageless vision: glare sensitivity, cataract amelioration and quality of vision currently available treatment for the challenging 50,000-patient population. Clin Interv Aging. 2009;4:31-50.

Babizhayev MA[1], Deyev AI,Efficacy of N-acetylcarnosine in the treatment of cataracts. Drugs R D. 2002;3(2):87-103

Guliaeva NV, Superoxide-scavenging activity of carnosine in the presence of copper and zinc ions. Biokhimiia 1987;52:1216-1220.

Hipkiss AR, Chana H. Carnosine protects proteins against methylglyoxal-mediated modifications. Biochem Biophys Res Commun 1998;248:28-32.

Schimel AM, Abraham L, N-acetylcysteine amide (NACA) prevents retinal degeneration by up-regulating reduced glutathione production and reversing lipid peroxidation. Am J Pathol. 2011 May;178(5):2032-4

Foods to prevent cataracts:

http://www.aoa.org/patients-and-public/caring-for-your-vision/nutrition/nutrition-and-cataracts?sso=y

Paul N Appleby, Naomi E Allen Diet, vegetarianism, and cataract risk, Am J Clin Nutr May 2011 vol. 93 no. 5 1128-1135

Paduru Yadagiri Reddy, Activation of sorbitol pathway in metabolic syndrome and increased susceptibility to cataract in Wistar-Obese rats Mol Vis. 2012; 18: 495–503.

Banditelli S1, Boldrini E Exp, A new approach against sugar cataract through aldose reductase inhibitors. Eye Res. 1999 Nov;69(5):533-8.

Çimen Karasu, Ahmet Cumaoğlu Interdiscip, Aldose reductase inhibitory activity and antioxidant capacity of pomegranate extracts Toxicol. Mar 2012; 5(1): 15–20.

Allen Taylor Paul F Jacques, Long-term intake of vitamins and carotenoids and odds of early age-related cortical and posterior subcapsular lens opacities; *The American Journal of Clinical Nutrition*, Volume 75, Issue 3, 1 March 2002, Pages 540–549

Hipkiss AR., Chapter 3 Carnosine and Its Possible Roles in Nutrition and Health. In: Steve LT, ed. *Advances in Food and Nutrition Research*. Vol Volume 57: Academic Press; 2009:87-154

Babizhayev MA, Failure to withstand oxidative stress induced by phospholipid hydroperoxides as a possible cause of the lens opacities in systemic diseases and ageing. Biochim Biophys Acta. Mar 1 1996;1315(2):87-99.

Christen W, Liu S, Glynn R, Gaziano M, Buring J. Dietary Carotenoids, Vitamins C and E, and Risk of Cataract in Women: A Prospective Study. Arch Ophthalmol. 2008;126(1):102-109

Seidler NW, Yeargans GS, Morgan TG. Carnosine disaggregates glycated [alpha]-crystallin: an in vitro study. Archives of Biochemistry and Biophysics. 2004;427(1):110-115.

Skin:

Kyung EunKim, DaehoCho Air pollution and skin diseases: Adverse effects of airborne particulate matter on various skin diseases Life Sciences Volume 152, 1 May 2016, Pages 126-134

Jean Krutmann, Pollution and skin: From epidemiological and mechanistic studies to clinical implications, Journal of Dermatological Science Volume 76, Issue 3, December 2014, Pages 163-168

Luisa Coderch, Ceramides and Skin Function, American Journal of Clinical Dermatology February 2003, Volume 4, Issue 2, pp 107–129

Rachel Grossman, The Role of Dimethylaminoethanol in Cosmetic Dermatology American Journal of Clinical Dermatology February 2005, Volume 6, Issue 1, pp 39–47

University of Illinois at Urbana-Champaign. "Exercise May Play Role In Reducing Inflammation In Damaged Skin Tissue." Science Daily. 4 December 2007

Murad Alam, Anne J. Walter, Association of Facial Exercise With the Appearance of Aging. JAMA Dermatology, 2018

Glenda Hall, MD, Estrogen and skin: The effects of estrogen, menopause, and hormone replacement therapy on the skin October 2005 Volume 53, Issue 4, Pages 555–568

ZhengYan, LiangHu Computer Vision Syndrome: A widely spreading but largely unknown epidemic among computer users, Computers in Human Behavior Volume 24, Issue 5, September 2008, Pages 2026-2042

Smita Agarwal, Dishanter Goe, Evaluation of the Factors which Contribute to the Ocular Complaints in Computer Users, J Clin Diagn Res. 2013 Feb; 7(2): 331–335.

Rosenfield M Computer vision syndrome: a review of ocular causes and potential treatments Ophthalmic Physiol Opt. 2011 Sep;31(5):502-15.

Made in the USA
Columbia, SC
23 November 2018